CW00430668

THE
HOMŒOPATHIC
AIDE- MEMOIRE

PETER COATS

THE C.W. DANIEL COMPANY LTD
1 Church Path
Saffron Walden
Essex, England

First published in Great Britain by
The C.W. Daniel Co. Ltd
1 Church Path
Saffron Walden
Essex
England

Completely Revised 1984

ISBN 0 850 32165 4

Set in Times by Simpson Typesetting,
Bishop's Stortford, Hertfordshire
and printed by D.R. Hillman Ltd
Frome, Somerset, England.

PREFACE

To ensure the best results it is necessary to have a Materia Medica in order that a comparison can be made between the patient's symptoms and the symptom picture of the chosen remedy.

They should be as near the same as possible.

"Materia Medica with Repertory" by Boericke is recommended as it is not too large.

Books the student should have are:—

"A Song of Symptoms" by Patersimilias.

"Leaders in Homoeopathic Therapeutics" by E. B. Nash, M.D.,

and,

"Homoeopathic Drug Pictures" by M. L. Tyler, M.D.

For a doctor,

"The Prescriber" by John H. Clark, M.D.

I wish to take this opportunity to thank all who, by their knowledge, have contributed to the making of this book.

CONTENTS

INTRODUCTION

Most books on Homoeopathy deal with both chronic and acute illness causing confusion to the inexperienced.

This booklet is designed to deal chiefly with acute conditions which last a comparatively short time.

Homoeopathic remedies deal quickly and safely with the troubles from which we suffer at various times, such as influenza, gastroenteritis, tainted food, etc.

To be a good Homoeopathic prescriber one has to have the brain of a detective and the eye of an artist.

One must search for symptoms like clues, note carefully the emotions and appearance of the patient: also any desires or aversions which are unusual.

Most of these will be found in Part 1 and should be carefully studied.

If the cause can be found it is a great help – weather conditions at the time should not be overlooked. It is necessary to point out that anything serious must be dealt with by a Doctor, preferably by a Homoeopathic Physician.

Dangerous symptoms could be the following, to mention a few:—

(1) Very high temperature.
(2) Pains in the chest.
(3) Pains in the abdomen with vomiting.
(4) A throat with a greyish-brown deposit.

I have included suggestions for pneumonia for the benefit of anyone who is unable to get a Doctor – they could also be useful in cases where antibiotics fail to work.

METHOD

Find three or four quite DEFINITE symptoms then look them up and you will discover by elimination a remedy common to each of them – if more than one remedy is found then search for another symptom to differentiate between them.

5

Those remedies in Capitals with an asterisk (*) before them are indicated more strongly than those without.

Those in ordinary print less so. Don't look only at those marked with an asterisk.

All in Capitals are important.

Here are some examples:—

Example 1.

The patient wakes at 2 a.m. feeling sick and ill – goes to the bathroom and vomits: this is followed by diarrhoea of a most offensive odour. The patient by now feels very weak and frightened with cold sweat. There is a desire for frequent sips of water as the mouth burns: the diarrhoea may also feel burning.

Your symptoms are:—

(1) *Time,* 2 a.m.
(2) *Vomiting* and diarrhoea.
(3) *Thirst,* for little and often.
(4) *Mouth* burning.
(5) *Emotions* – Fear.

Common to these symptoms is ARS: The name of the illness is not important. The doses should be given every quarter of an hour in severe cases and every half-hour in less severe cases for the first three doses – then every four hours if necessary.

Normally give the 6 potency or, if very ill, the 30. If only one strength is kept then the 12 will probably be the most useful, but for the inexperienced use the 6 only.

Example 2.

The patient wakes feeling very ill – on taking the temperature at about 10 a.m. it is found to be high. The eyes are heavy lidded and the eyeballs sore – cannot stand any bright light. There is a severe headache often starting at the back and settling over one eye. The back of the neck feels slightly stiff and sore. There are bruised pains in the limbs. The patient feels miserable with shivers up and down the back and wants to be left alone – there may be trembling. There is usually NO THIRST. It was noted that the weather was humid (See "Cause"). There are likely to be common cold symptoms as well.

Your symptoms are:—

(1) *Alone*. Wishes to be left alone.
(2) *Eyes*. Eyeballs sore.
(3) *Thirst*. Thirstless during fever.
(4) *Headache*. Starting at back of head and settling over one eye.
(5) *Pains*. Sore, bruised.
(6) *Sensitivity*. Light aggravates.

The remedy is GEL: The dosage would be the 12 or 30 potency every two hours for the first three doses, then four hourly. After the temperature is normal at night, give another three doses every four hours.

This is a typical picture of influenza but note NOT every influenza – always go by the symptoms.

Example 3.

A young patient of 6 years lies very still on her right side (her only comfortable position). Both food and drink are vomited a few minutes after swallowing. In spite of this she wants only very cold water. (See "Hot and Cold"). When questioned, replies after a long pause and very slowly. She has a temperature and a headache across the forehead. It is noticed she had changed her position in bed with her head at the foot to avoid the direct light from the window.

Your symptoms are:—

(1) *Sides*. Worse on the left.
(2) *Vomiting*. After water becomes warm in stomach.
(3) *Answers*. Slowly.
(4) *Headache*. Forehead.
(5) *Motion* – inactive – lethargic.
(6) *Sensitivity*. Light aggravates.

The remedy here is PHO: Dose, the 6 potency every half-hour for three doses – then every four hours only if required.

Example 4.

This patient has a fairly high temperature – the body is slightly moist – the eyes have the pupils much enlarged. There is a throbbing headache at the temples – the tongue is bright red and so is the throat. The cheeks are red and burning hot to touch. There can be delirium, sometimes quite violent – slightest jar hurts.

Your symptoms are:—

(1) *Facial Appearance.* Pupils of eyes enlarged, also cheeks burning hot to touch.
(2) *Headache.* Temples throb.
(3) *Throat,* colour – bright red.
(4) *Tongue.* Bright red or like a strawberry.
(5) *Sensitivity.* To jar on stepping hard.

Your remedy is BELL: Dose every hour for first 3 doses, then every four hours as required. The 12 potency.

I have mentioned six symptoms in each of these examples, but three or four that you are quite certain about will do.

If there is no improvement at all after three doses you will probably have chosen the wrong remedy.

Strength or Potency

The potency is the strength of the remedy and is denoted by a number after the name. (The names are all abbreviated to save space, such as BELL: for BELLADONNA). The higher the number the greater the strength and the more accurate one must be. For beginners and children the 6, or in some instances the 12, are recommended. More severe cases may require the 30 and very occasionally the 200, but only by someone with experience.

Repetition

A general rule is that the more rapid the disease the more often you must repeat the dose – for instance in violent diarrhoea and vomiting, every quarter of an hour – or in influenza every 2 hours for the first 3 doses and then four hourly as required – see Examples 1 and 2 – for lumbago perhaps only three doses might be required such as Rhus-t 12, night, morning, night.

Always *STOP* the medicine as soon as there is a marked improvement – this is MOST important.

Exceptions are true influenza and pneumonia, where it is advisable to continue the remedy for 2 or 3 doses at four hourly intervals after the temperature is normal in the evening.

Method of Taking

It is best to take the remedy on a relatively empty stomach. Allow the pills or tablet to dissolve slowly on the tongue – no accompanying drink of water is necessary. The mouth should be clean and free of toothpaste or any other strong smelling substance.

It is advisable to avoid drinking coffee or taking ordinary medicines such as aspirin while treatment is in progress.

Dosage

The remedies are made up in either little pills or tablets, also in tiny granules: the latter dissolve quickly in water and are useful for babies – for children under seven years one pill – for adults two pills or if tablets are used, one for adults. When granules are employed for a baby, use the equivalent amount of a crushed tablet and dissolve in three tablespoonfuls of cold water. Administer in teaspoonful doses – do not handle the pills or leave the bottles uncapped. The bottles should be kept in a drawer that has no smell: as moth balls, strong perfumes or camphorated oil etc., can completely destroy their effectiveness. Finally, buy your medicines from a reliable source.

IMPORTANT

All treatment should be under proper medical

surveillance except for minor ailments

of a not serious nature.

Editor

ALONE or COMPANY

WISHES TO BE ALONE
*ANAC: ANT-c: *BAR-c: Bell: Bry: Cact: Carb-an: Carb-v: CHIN: FER: FER-p: *GEL: *IGN: Iod: LACH: Led: Lyc: Nat-c: *NAT-m: NUX-v: Rhus-t: SEP: Stan: Sul: Thu:

DESIRES COMPANY
*ACON: ANT-t: AP: *ARG-n: *ARS: *BISM: CALC-c: Clem: Con: Dros: Hep: *KALI-c: KALI-p: *LAC-c: Lyc: *PHO: *PULS: SEP: *STRAM: Vera-a:

Note: Lyc: Likes someone within call.
Bry: Gets angry if disturbed.

ANSWERS

ANSWERS SLOWLY
ANAC: *BAPT: CARB-v: COCCL: CON: Gel: HELL: KALI-bi: *MERC: NUX-m: *PH-ac: *PHO: Rhus-t: SUL: THU: Zn:

REFUSES TO ANSWER
AGAR: ARN: CHIN: CIMIC: Glo: HELL: HYOS: NUX-v: *PHO: STRAM: *SUL: Sul-ac: VER-a:

CAUSE

COLD, WET WEATHER, DAMP ROOMS. GETTING SOAKED.
*AM-c: *ANT-c: ANT-t: *ARS: *CALC-c: CIMIC: *DUL: KALI-io: *NUX-m: *NAT-s: *PULS: RHOD: *RHUS-t: SEP: *SIL: *TUB:

10

DRY, CLEAR COLD
*ACO: Ars: *ASAR: Bry: *CAUST: *HEP: Ip:
*KALI-c: *NUX-v: Sabad: Sil: Spig: Spong:

FROST, SNOW AIR
AGAR: Ars: CALC-c: Carb-v: Caust: *CON:
Form: Lyc: Mag-m: Nit-ac: Nux-v: Petr: Pho:
PH-ac: PULS: Rhus-t: *SEP: SIL: SUL: Syph: Urt-u: Vib-o:

HUMID, WARM, WET
*CARB-v: *GEL: IOD: KALI-bi: *LACH: *NAT-s:
Puls: SIL:

SUMMER, HOT WEATHER
AETH: ALUM: Alo: *ANT-c: BELL: BRY:
CARB-s: CARB-v: Chion: *FLAC-ac: Gel: IOD:
Iris: GUAJ: KALI-bi: LACH: LYC: NAT-c: NAT-m:
NUX-v: *POD: PULS: SABI: SEL: Thu: Ver-v:

SUN, OVER-EXPOSURE. FIRE HEAT.
ACON: AGAR: *ANT-c: *BELL: BRY: Carb-v:
GEL: *GLO: KALI-c: LACH: Merc: *NAT-c:
*NAT-m: NUX-v: *OP: PULS: *SEL: Sul: Ther:
Ver-v:

WIND – COLD NORTH EAST
*ACON: ARS: *BELL: *BRY: Caust: Cham:
*HEP: Kali-bi: *NUX-v: Sep: Sil: SPIG: *SPONG:

WINDY
ACO: Ars: *BELL: Calc-c: Calc-p: Caps: *CHAM:
CHIN: Colch: Colo: *HEP: Kali-c: Lach: *LYC:
*NUX-v: *PHO: Ph-ac: *PULS: *RHOD: RHUS-t:
Samb: Sele: *SIL: SPONG: Stro: Squil: *SUL:

CHANGE FROM COLD TO WARM
*BRY: CHEL: FER: *KALI-s: LACH: LYC:
NAT-m: NAT-s: *PSOR: PULS: *SUL: *TUB:

CHILLED WHILE HOT – EATING ICES – BATHING ETC.
ACO: BELL: *BELS: HEP: NUX-v: Pho: RHUS-t:
Sil:

OVER-INDULGENCE IN:

Alcohol	NUX-v:
Beer	KALI-bi:
Food	BRY: Carb-vi: NUX-v:
New potatoes	NAT-s:
Pastry, cream, fats	PULS:
Sweets or Sugar	NAT-p:
Bad fish and shell fish	ARS: CARB-v:
Bad food	*ARS:
Iced drinks while hot	BELS:
Upset by cabbage, * beans, peas*	BRY: LYC:
Inability to digest milk	AETHUSA: SIL

BRUISE, SHOCK, ACCIDENT
*ARN:

BLOW ON BREAST (Woman)
*BELS:

BLOW ON EYE
LED: SYMP:

CRUSHED FINGERS OR TOES
*HYPR:

FALL ON TAIL (Coccyx)
*HYPR:

OVER PHYSICAL EXERTION
*ARN: Ars: Bels: Bry: Calc-c: NAT-c: Nat-m: Nux-v:
*RHUS-t: *RUT: Staph: Sul:

SWELLING OF TONGUE OR THROAT
obstructing breathing (such as a sting in the mouth)
*API:

VERY LONG RETARDED MENTAL SHOCK
NAT-m:

VERY LONG RETARDED PHYSICAL SHOCK
OP:

Note: SUL-ac: if required, follows ARN: well in bruises
of soft parts.
CON: in bruises of glands and
RUT: in bruises of bones.
NAT-s 30: pain in head long after injury 3 times a
day for some time.

EMOTIONS

ANTICIPATION
*ARG-n: Ars: Carb-v: *GEL: Lyc: Plb: Ph-ac: SIL:

FASTIDIOUS
Anac: *ARS: Graph: *Nat-s: *NUX-v: Pho: Plat:
Sep: Sil:

FEAR
*ACO: *ARG-n: *ARS: *AUR: Bapt: *BELL:
*BOR: BRY: *CALC-c: *CALC-p: *CARB-v:
Caust: *DIG: Gel: Grap: *IGN: *LACH: *LYC:
NAT-m: NIT-ac: *NUX-v: OP: *PHO: *PULS:
SEP: STRA: SUL: VER-a:

FEAR OF ANIMALS
*CHIN: TUB:

FEAR OF CROWDS
*ACO: *ARG-n: Aur: Gel: *NAT-m: Puls:

FEAR OF THE DARK
ACON: *CALC-c: CARB-v: CAUST: CUPR:
LYC: PHO: *PULS: *STRAM: (compare "Wishes
Company").

FEAR OF ROBBERS
Arg-n: *ARS: Ign: NAT-m: Lach: Merc: Pho:

FEAR OF THUNDER
Lyc: Nat-c: *PHO:

FEARS he has some TERRIBLE DISEASE
Lil-t: Kali-c: Pho: Nit-ac: Sep:

13

GRIEF

AUR: CAUS: *IGN: Lach: Lyc: Nat-m: PH-ac: PULS: STAP:

INDIFFERENCE AND APATHY

Ap: Arn: Bapt: CALC-c: Carb-v: Chin: Con: Gel: *HELL: Ign: Nat-c: Nat-m: OP: PHO: *PH-ac: Plat: *PULS: *SEP: Stap: Sul: Tab:

IRRITABLE

*ACO: ANT-c: APIS: *ARS: *BRY: *CALC-c: Calc-p: *CHAM: CINA: COLO: *HEP: IGN: *KALI-c: KALI-p: *LYC: *NAT-m: *NIT-ac: *NUX-v: Pho: *SEP: STAP: *SUL: etc.,

JEALOUSY

Lach: Hyo: Api: Calc-s: Nux-v: Puls: Stram:

RUDENESS OR INDIGNATION

*STAP:

STUBBORN

ACON: *ALU: *ARG-n: *BELL: BRY: *CALC-c: *CHAM: CHIN: *NUX-v: SIL: SUL: TARENT: TUB: etc.,

TEARFUL

AETH: *AP: AUR: BEL: *CACT: *CALC-c: *CAUS: CHAM: *GRAP: *IGN: *LYC: *NAT-m: *NUX-m: Pho: *PLAT: *PULS: *RHUS-t: *SEP: *SUL: *VER-a: etc.,

Note

DREAD OF AN ORDEAL, such as stage fright, exam-funk or enclosed places, heights, etc., ARG-n.

SHAKING WITH APPREHENSION before an event, such as an important interview: GEL:

SUDDEN FRIGHT OR FEAR, either mental or physical: ACO:

INABILITY TO CONCENTRATE (Children), Aeth-c: Bar-c:

CLAUSTROPHOBIA in tube trains, tunnels, etc.,
ARG-n: NAT-m:

FACIAL APPEARANCE

EYELIDS, HEAVY, FALLING
BAP: Caus: Cham: Coccl: Con: *GEL: *KALI-p:
Nux-v: Rhus-t: SEP: Spi: Ver-a:

PUPILS OF EYES ENLARGED
AGAR: *BELL: Bry: GEL: HYOS: STRAM: CIC:
HELL:

PUPILS CONTRACTED
*ACON: AP: PHO: OP:

CHEEKS BURNING, HOT TO TOUCH
*BELL: CALC-c: CHAM: *CINA: CLEM: FER:
*FER-p: *GEL: Merc: NUX-v:

GLOWING RED
ACON: *BELL: *CHAM: Chin: *CINA: FER:
IGN: Hep: Lyc: Nux-v: Pho: PULS: Sul:

RED BECOMES DEATHLY PALE ON RISING
*ACON: Ver-a:

ONE CHEEK PALE THE OTHER RED
ACON: ARN: Bar-c: *CHAM: CINA: *IP: LACH:
NUX-v: PHO: PULS: Ran-b: Spig: Sul:

COLD SWEAT ON FACE
ANT-t: *ARS: *CACT: *CARB-v: *CINA:
*MERC-c: NUX-v: *SPONG: TAB: *VER-a:

DARK, DUSKY RED, BESOTTED LOOKING
Arn: *BAP: Bry: Crot-h: *GEL: Hyo: *OP: Stram:

PALE AROUND MOUTH AND NOSE
Cina: PHO:

HEAT WITH HEADACHE
CHIN-s: GLON: Rumx: SPONG:

YELLOW FACE
ARS: BRY: CARB-v: *CARD-m: *CHEL:
*CHIN: FER: *LYC: *MERC: *NUX-v: *PLB:
POD: *SEP: SUL:

FACE SWOLLEN
Am-m: AP: *ARS: *BELL: BRY: Cham: Kali-c:
LYC: *MERC: NUX-v: Op: Pho: RHUS-t: Stram:

BLUISH
Aco: ARS: Bell: *CUP: Ip: LACH: Op: VER-a:
VER-v:

REDDISH YELLOW
*CHEL: Gel: Lach: *NUX-v:

DEATHLY COLD (COLLAPSED)
ARS: *CARB-v: VER-a: (These three in high
potency).

HEADACHES

FOREHEAD
ACO: AM-c: ARS: *BELL: Berb: BISM: *BRY:
CAPS: Chin: COCCL: Fer-p: Gel: HEP: HYDR:
Ign: KALI-bi: Lach: Lyc: MERC: NAT-m: *NUX-v:
PHO: Phyt: Pru-s: PULS: RHUS-T: SABAD: Sep:
Sil: SPIG: SUL: Thu: Ver-a: VIOLA-o:

TOP OF HEAD (vertex)
Ap: Brom: CACT: Calc-c: CALC-p: Carb-a: Caus:
*CIMIC: Glo: Hypr: *LACH: Lyc: Men: NIT-ac:
Pho: PH-ac: RAN-ac: *SIL: *SUL: VER-a:

BACK OF HEAD AND NAPE (occiput)
Agar: AP: Arn: BELL: BRY: Calc-c: CARB-v:
Caul: Caust: Chin: *CIMIC: Coccl: *EUP-pf:
*GEL: Glon: IGN: Lachn: *NAT-s: NUX-v: Onos:
PETR: PHYT: RHUS-t: Sanic: Sep: *SIL: SUL:
Ver-v: Zn:

SIDES
Anac: Arg-n: *BELL: *CHIN: Cycl: GLO: Kali-c:
KALI-p: Kre: Nux-m: Nux-v: Par: Ph-ac: Plat:
PULS: Rhus-t: Sabi: SPIG: Thu: Verb: Zn: etc.,

TEMPLES THROB
Arg-n: FER-p: *BELL: Gel: GLO: PYRO: Zn-chr:

OVER EYES
Arn: ARS: Bar-c: BELL: Bism: *BRY: CARB-v:
Cad: Chel: CHIN-s: *GEL: HYDR: Iris: KALI-bi:
*LACH: Lil-t: Lyc: Naj: *NAT-m: *NUX-v: PHO:
PULS: SABAD: Sang: *SIL: *SPIG: Zn:

THROBBING, HAMMERING
Aco: *BELL: BRY: Cact: *CAD-s: Calc-c: *CHIN:
Coccl: EUP-pf: *FER-p: GLO: *LACH: Laur:
LYC: MELLI: *NAT-m: *PYRO: SANG: Sep: SIL:
Stap: Sul:

STARTING LOW AT BACK OF HEAD AND SETTLING OVER ONE EYE
Arg-n: BELL: CALC-c: Carb-v: CIMIC: *GEL:
GLO: KALI-bi: Lac-c: Lach: Lil-t: Onos: PAR:
Petr: Pho: Sabad: *SANG: SARS: Sep: *SIL: SPIG:
Sul: VER-v:

SCHOOL CHILDREN
Calc-c: *CALC-p: Nat-m: PH-ac: Puls:

TELEVISION HEADACHE
CALC-p:

HEAT AND COLD

HOT APPLICATIONS RELIEVE
*ARS: (except head) BELL: CALC-fl: Caus: Cham:
Chin: Clem: Coccl: Dros: *GRAPH: *HEP: Hyo:
KALI-bi: *KALI-c: Lyc: Mag-c: *MAG-p: MERC:
Nat-c: Nux-m: *NUX-v: Rhod: *RHUS-t: Rumx:
SAMB: Scil: Sep: *SIL: *STRO: Sul: Zn:

COLD APPLICATION RELIEVES
ACO: AP: ARG-n: *ARS: (head only) Asar: AUR:
BRY: Calc-c: *CHAM: Dros: Fer: Fer-p: FLU-ac:
Guai: *IOD: Kali-s: LED: *LYC: Merc: Mur-ac:
NAT-m: OP: *PULS: Phyt: Rhus-t: Sabi: Sec-c:
Spig: *SUL: Tab:

COLD AIR AGGRAVATES
*AGAR: *ALL-c: *ARS: (except head) AUR: Bry: CALC-c: *CALC-p: *CAUST: *CIMIC: Coloc: *DULC: Fer-p: Graph: *HEP: Kali-bi: *KALI-c: LYC: *MAG-p: NUX-m: *NUX-v: Pho: *RHOD: *RHUS-t: *RUMX: *SABAD: *SEP: *SIL: (Compare under "Cause").

UNCOVERING AGGRAVATES
(See under "Sensitivity to Draughts").

WARM ROOM AGGRAVATES
Ant-c: *ANT-t: *AP: ARG-n: BRY: *CALC-s: *CARB-v: CROC: Dros: *GRAP: *IOD: IP: KALI-io: *KALI-s: *LACH: LED: LYC: MERC-i-f: NAT-c: NAT-s: OP: *PULS: Pyrog: SABI: *SEC-c: *SENG: SPONG: *SUL: TUB: Thu: VER-a:

HEAT OF FIRE RELIEVES
*ARS: DULC: *HEP: IGN: *MAG-p: NUX-m: *NUX-v: *RHUS-t: *SIL:

HEAT OF SUN OR FIRE AGGRAVATES
(See under "Cause").

Note: ARS: and PHO: Like a cool head and a warm body. In the stomach symptoms of PHO: Cold drinks and foods are preferred but often vomited after a few minutes.

INSPIRING COLD AIR AGGRAVATES
*ACO: *AM-c: Aesc: Ars: CARB-v: *CAUS: CIMIC: Cist: *HEP: Hyds: HYO: IGN: *MERC: Nat-s: Nit-ac: NUX-v: *RUMX: SABAD: Seneg: Sep: *SPONG:

DESIRES COOL FRESH AIR
Alu: AP: ARG-n: ARS: AUR: *CARB-v: Croc: Glo: Iod: KALI-io: *KALI-s: *LACH: Lil-t: LYC: Mag-c: MAG-m: NAT-s: Op: *PULS: Rhus-t: Sabad: *SUL: Tub:

MOTION AND INACTIVE

MOVEMENTS AGGRAVATE
*ANT-t: Arn: *BELL: *BISM: *BRY: *CAD-s:
Calc-c: *CHEL: *CHIN: *COCCL: *COLOC:
*COLCH: EUP-pf: FER-p: Kali-c: *LED: *MERC:
Nat-m: Nit-ac: *NUX-v: Pho: *SIL: SPIG: *SUL:
Ver-a:

MOVEMENT RELIEVES
Ant-t: Arg-n: Ars: *AUR: *CAPS: *CON: *CYC:
*DUL: *EUPHOR: *FER: Fer-p: Flu-ac: KALI-c:
KALI-io: KRE: *LYC: MAG-c: MAG-m: MERC:
*PYROG: *PULS: *RHOD: *RHUS-t: *SABAD:
SAMB: SEP: *SUL: TARENT: *TARX: *VAL:
ZN:

FIRST MOVEMENT AGGRAVATES BUT CONTINUED MOVEMENT TEMPORARILY IMPROVES
Bap: CALC-fl: *CAPS: CAUS: *CON: *EUPHOR:
FER: *LYC: PHO: *PULS: Pyr: *RHUS-t: SAMB:
Sep: (Compare "Restless").

BREATHING DEEPLY AGGRAVATES
*ACO: ARN: *BOR: *BRY: *CALC-c: Caus:
CHEL: *KALI-c: Pho: Ran-b: Rhus-t: Rumx: Sabi:
Sang: Scil: Spig: *SQUIL: Sul:

SLOW GENTLE MOVEMENT RELIEVES
Agar: Alu: Amb: AUR: Colo: *FER: Glo: KALI-p:
Mag-m: *PULS: TARN:

ACT OF SITTING-UP AGGRAVATES
*ACO: *BELL: *BRY: CAD-s: CHEL: *COCCL:
*DIG: FER: IGN: LYC: MERC-i-f: NAT-m: NIT-
ac: *NUX-v: *OP: PHO: PHYT: PULS: *RHUS-t:
*SIL: *SUL:

INACTIVE, LETHARGIC
All-c: Ant-t: ARN: ARS: BAP: Bar-m: Cald: Calc-
c: HELL: Lac-d: NUX-v: Old: *OP: *PHO: *PH-ac:
Rad: *SEP: STRA: SUL: Thry: Zn:

PATIENT "MUST LIE DOWN"
ACO: ALU: Ap: Aran: Ars: Bap: Bar-m: *BRY:
CAD-s: Cald: Carb-s: CHAM: COCCL: Fer: Fer-p:
*GEL: Kali-bi: Kali-s: Kali-c: LACH: NAT-sal:
*NUX-v: PIC-ac: *RHUS-t: SEP: *SELE: SIL:
STAN:

MOUTH

BURNING – RAW – SMARTING
ARS: Arum-t: BELL: BOR: Cham: GEL: Iris:
Med: Mez: Puls: Sang: Sep: Sul: Sul-io:

DRYNESS, WITH GREAT THIRST
Acon: ARS: BRY: Pod: Pho-ac: Rhus-t: Sul: Ver-a:

DRY BUT NOT THIRSTY
All-c: *AP: BAPT: Bell: BRY: Calad: COCCL:
Dulc: Kali-c: Lac-c: Lach: *LYC: *NUX-m: NUX-v:
Paris: *PULS: Pyro: Sabad: SIL: Spig: Stram:

Note: BRY: usually has great thirst.

SALIVA INCREASED
AM-c: BAR-c: *BOR: Dulc: FL-ac: IOD: IP:
KALI-c: LYSS: *MERC: *MERC-c: *MERC-i-r:
*NAT-m: NIT-ac: NUX-v: PHO: Plb: PULS: Rhus-t:
STRAM: *VER-a: Zn:

SALIVA THICK
ARS: BERB: *CHEL: *KALI-bi: *LACH: *LYSS:
*MERC: *MERC-c: NUX-m: Phyt: PULS: Stram:

TASTE BAD, PUTRID
Anac: ARN: Calc-c: Caps: *GEL: MERC: Nat-s:
*NUX-v: *PULS: Psor: *PYRO: RHUS-t: Stan:
Sul: Syph: Vario:

TASTE BITTER
*ACO: ANT-c: *ARS: *BRY: CARB-v: *CHEL:
*CHIN: COLOC: LYC: *MERC: NAT-m: *NUX-v:
*PULS: SEP: *SUL: VER-a: etc.,

GREASY, FATTY
ALU: Asaf: Caus: Iris: Kali-p: Petr: *PULS: Tril:

METALLIC
    COCCL: Cup: Iod: Kali-bi: *MERC: NAT-c: Nux-v:
    RHUS-t: Seneg: Thry: Vario: Zn-ar:

SALTY
    ARS: Con: Kali-bi: Kali-io: Lyc: MERC: Merc-c:
    *NAT-m: Pho: Puls: SEP:

ULCERS (Aphthae)
    *ARS: Bap: *BOR: Iod: Kali-bi: Kali-io: Lach:
    *MERC: Merc-c: Mur-ac: *NIT-ac: Nux-v: Rhus-t:
    SUL: SUL-ac: *THU: Mag-c:6,

LOSS OF TASTE AND SMELL
    Anac: *BELL: Crot-t: Just: MAG-m: *NAT-m:
    *PHOS: *PULS: Sil:

TOBACCO TASTES BITTER
    Camph: *CHIN: COCCL: EUPHR: Nat-m:
    SPONG:

HERPES ON LIPS – SMALL AND HARD
    Calc-fl:

HERPES ROUND THE MOUTH
    Nat-m: Ran-b: Rhus-t:

TONGUE

A slightly coated Tongue is not a useful symptom.
Various colours produced by highly coloured foods and
drinks can be misleading.

BROWNISH
    Am-c: Ant-t: ARS: Bapt: BRY: Cup-ar: Echin:
    Hyos: Med: MERC-cy: Mur-ac: Nat-s: Phos: Sec:
    Viper:

BROWNISH DRY
    AIL: Ant-t: ARS: BAPT: BRY: Carb-v: Kali-p:
    LACH: RHUS-t: Spong:

BROWN CENTRE
    BAPT: Pho: Plb:

DRY
ACON: ARS: BELL: BRY: Calc-c: GEL: Kali-p:
LACH: MUR-ac: NUX-m: PARIS: Pho: Pyro:
*RHUS-t: Sul: Tereb: VER-v:

**FLABBY, WET, WITH IMPRINTS OF TEETH
AROUND EDGES**
Ars: Chel: HYDR: Kali-bi: Merc-c: MERC-d:
*MERC: Nat-p: POD: Pyro: RHUS-t: Sanic: Stram:

GREY
Kali-m:

GREENISH GREY
Kali-s: *NAT-s: NIT-ac: Plb:

RED – BRIGHT
Acon: *AP: *ARS: *BELL: GEL: Hyo: KALI-bi:
Lach: MERC: *PHO: *RHUS-t:

RED EDGES
*ARS: BELL: *CHEL: *MERC: *SUL:

RED EDGES WITH WHITE CENTRE
BELL: LAC-c: RHUS-t:

RED TIP
*ARS: LACH: LYC: Merc-i-r: NIT-ac: *PHYT:
*RHUS-t: *SUL:

STRAWBERRY
*BELL:

TYPHOID, DARK STREAK IN CENTRE
Arn: Bapt: Mur-ac:

YELLOW – DIRTY THICK COATING
BAPT: Bry: *CHEL: CHIN: *GEL: Hyds: KALI-bi:
Kali-p: *MERC: MERC-i-f: *NAT-p: Nat-s: NUX-v:
NUX-m: Phyt: PULS: *RHUS-t: *SPIG: SUL:

PATCHY, LIKE A MAP
ARS: Dul: Hydr: KALI-bi: Kali-m: LACH: Merc:
MERC-c: *NAT-m: NIT-ac: Ran-sc: RHUS-t: Sep:
TARX: Tub:

WHITE LIKE WHITEWASH
*ANT-c: ANT-t: ARS: SUL: NUX-v:

PAIN, PRESSURE AND DIRECTION

ACHING, BONE-BREAKING PAINS
Coccl: PYRO: *EUP-pf:

BURSTING PAINS, are found in most leading remedies –
(Compare under "Sensations").

BURSTING OR SPLITTING
Asaf: *BELL: *BRY: Calc-c: Caust: CHIN: Eup-pf:
Glo: Ham: Ign: Kali-m: Lac-c: Lil-t: Lyc: MERC:
*NAT-m: Nit-ac: *NUX-v: Rat: Sep: Sil: Spig: Stan:
Sul: *VIP:

CRAMP AND COLIC
BELL: Cact: *CALC-c: Caus: CHAM: CHIN:
Coccl: *COLO: *CUP: DIO: GRAP: IGN: Lach:
LYC: Mag-m: *MAG-p: Nat-m: Nit-ac: *NUX-v:
PLAT: Plb: *PULS: Sil: *SUL: VER-a: Vib: Zn:

CRAMP IN MUSCLES
Anac: Bell: *CALC-c: CHIN: Cina: CON: *CUP:
*CUP-ar: Lyc: *MAG-p: Merc: *NUX-v: Plat: Sep:
Tab:

GROWING PAINS IN JOINTS
PH-ac:

CUTTING
Aco: *BELL: Bry: CALC-c: Calc-p: Calc-s:
CANTH: *COLO: CON: Dio: Gamb: Hyo: *KALI-c:
KALI-m: LYC: Merc: Nat-c: Nat-m: Nit-ac:
*NUX-v: Petr: Plan: POLY: PULS: Rat: Rumx:
Sabl: Sil: Staph: SUL: Tell: Ver-a: Zn:

BONE PAINS
AUR: Asaf: EUP-pf: MERC-s:

SHOOTING
Aco: AGAR: Alu: Arg-n: Ars: *BELL: BERB:
*CIMIC: COLO: Cup: CIO: FER: Hyd-ac: Hyo:
*HYP: KALI-bi: KALI-c: Kalm: Lyc: Mag-c: Mag-m:

MAG-p: NIT-ac: Nux-v: Ox-ac: Paeo: Plb: Pru-s: Rad: Ran-b: Rhus-t: Sabi: Sec-c: SPIG: *SUL: Ver-a: Xan: Zn:

STABBING OR STITCHING

ACON: Bell: BERB: BOR: *BRY: CANTH: CHEL: CHIN: IGN: *KALI-c: LACH: LED: MERC: MERC-c: NAT-s: NIT-ac: *PHO: PLB: PULS: *RAN-b: Rhus-t: SEP: SIL: *SPIG: SQUIL: Staph: Sul: Thuj: etc.,

BURNING, STINGING, SMARTING

Ant-c: *AP: ARUM-t: ARS: BERB: Bry: *CANTH: Con: Caps: Dul: EQUIS: GLO: Iris: Kali-c: Lyc: Merc: Mez: Nit-ac: Nux-v: PHO: Ph-ac: Puls: Rhus-t: Sabi: SEP: *SIL: Stap: SUL: Tarn: URT-u: Zn:

SORE – BRUISED

AP: *ARN: Aur: BAP: BELL: BERB: *BRY: *CAPS: Canth: CARB-v: CAUS: CHIN: Cimic: CON: DROS: *EUP-pf: *GEL: Hep: LACH: Lyc: NAT-m: NIT-ac: *NUX-v: Pho: Phyt: PULS: *PYRO: Ran-b: *RHUS-t: *RUT: *SIL: SUL: Zn:

SPLINTER OR PRICKING FEELING OF SHARP STICKS

(See under "Sensations").

Note: ARN: has a bruised soreness.

> *CAUS:* has more a rawness; mostly of mucous surfaces.

> *RHUS-t:* has an aching sprained soreness in muscles and tendons.

THROBBING – PULSATING

ANT-t: ACO: *BELL: Bry: CAD-s: *CALC-c: CARB-v: Chin: COCCL: Con: EUP-pf: *FER: *GLO: LACH: *GRAPH: KALI-c: LYC: NAT-m: PHO: *PULS: *PYRO: SEP: SABI: Sang: SIL: SUL: Verv-v: Zn:

In Blood Vessels, *BELL: *GLO:

In Glands, Calc-c: *CON: Kali-c: *MERC: Pho

PRESSURE AGGRAVATES; ALSO WORSE LYING ON PAINFUL SIDE

Acon: *AGAR: *AP: Ars: *BAR-c: Colad: Calc-c: CARB-v: *CINA: *HEP: *IOD: *LACH: *LYC: MERC-c: NAT-m: NUX-v: *SIL: Stap:

PRESSURE RELIEVES

AM-c: ARG-n: *BRY: CHEL: *CHIN: *COLO: *CON: *DROS: Dul: Ign: *MAG-m: *MAG-p: *NAT-c: *PLB: *PULS: RHUS-t: SEP: *SIL: SPI: STAN:

HARD PRESSURE RELIEVES

CHIN: *COIO: LACH: MAG-p: NUX-v: Plb: Sang: Zn:

TOUCH AGGRAVATES, BUT HARD PRESSURE RELIEVES

Bell: CASTR: CHIN: Ign: LACH: NUX-v: Plb:

SLIGHT TOUCH AGGRAVATES

Aco: Ap: Ars: *BELL: *CHEL: *CHIN: COLCH: GEL: *HEP: IGN: *LACH: Mag-m: *MERC: MEZ: NIT-ac: *NUX-v: PHO: STAN:

DIRECTION

ASCENDING. Aco: ASAF: BELL: Clac-c: Con: Gel: GLO: *IGN: *LACH: LED: Naj: *PHO: PULS: Sabad: *SANG: *SEP: *SIL: SUL: Zn:

BACKWARD. BELL: BRY: *CHEL: Con: Cup: Gel: KALI-bi: Kali-c: Lil-t: LYC: MERC: Nat-m: Par: Pho: Pru-sp: Puls: SEP: Spi: *SUL:

CROSSWISE. Bell: Berb: Calc-c: CHEL: CHIN: Fer: Hell: Ip: Kali-bi: Kali-m: LAC-c: Rad: Sep: Sil: SUL: Val: Ver-a: Zn:

CROSSWISE ALTERNATING. Agar: Bell: Cimic: COCCL: Croc: Glo: IGN: *LAC-c: Lach: *LYC: PHO: PULS: *SUL:

DIAGONAL. AGAR: ALU: Amb: Ap: Bor: Kali-bi:

25

KALM: Lach: Lyc: MANG: Murx: Nat-c: Nux-v: PHO: *RHUS-t: Stict: SUL-ac: Tarx:

DOWNWARD. Alo: Arn: Aur: Bar-c: BERB: Bor: Bry: Caps: Cic: Coff: Hyp: KALM: Lach: Latro: LYC: Par-b: Puls: Rhod: Rhus-t: Sanic: Selen: Zn:

FORWARD. Berb: Bry: Carb-v: GEL: LAC-c: SABI: SANG: Sep: Sil: *SPIG:

OUTWARDS. ASAF: Bell: Berb: Bry: Chin: Con: Hyp: Ign: Kali-bi: Kali-m: Kalm: Latro: Lith: Pru-s: Sep: Sil: Sul: VAL: Zn:

RADIATING. Agar: Arg-m: Ars: Bab: *BERB: Caps: Caus: Cham: Cimic: *COLO: *CUP: *DIO: Gel: Hep: Kali-bi: Kali-c: Kali-m: Kalm: Lach: Latro: Lyc: Mag-p: *MERC: Mez: Nit-ac: NUX-v: Phyt: Plat: Plb: Sec-c: Sil: Spig: Tell: Xan:

UP AND DOWN _ FALLING AND RISING SENSATION. Ars: Bap: Bry: Calc-c: Cimic: Eup-pf: GEL: GLO: Kali-c: Lach: Lil-t: Lyc: Osm: PHO: PLB: Pod: SUL: VER-a:

WANDERING, SHIFTING. Amb: Arn: Asaf: Ben-ac: Berb: Calc-p: CAUL: Cimic: Colch: Croc: Fer: Gel: *KALI-bi: Kali-m: Kali-n: *KALI-s: Kalm: *LAC-c: *LED: Mag-c: Mag-p: Merc-i-r: Nux-m: Pall: Plan: Poly: Pru-s: *PULS: Rad: Rhod: Rhus-t: Sep: Sil: Stro: Tab: Thu: Tub: VAL: (Compare "Sides Alternating").

POSTURE

BENDING FORWARD OR DOUBLING-UP RELIEVES
Aco: Beryl: CALC-c: Caps: Caus: Cham: Chin:
Cimic: *COLO: Graph: KALI-c: Lyc: Mag-m:
*MAG-p: Merc: Par-b: Puls: RHE: RHUS-t: Sec-c:
SEP: SUL: Thu:

BENDING BACKWARD RELIEVES
Alet: ALU: *ANT-t: Arn: Bell: Bism: CALC-c:
*DIOS: GUAI: Hep: IGN: Lyc: NUX-v: PULS:
Rhus-t: Sabi: SEC-c:

LYING AGGRAVATES
AMB: ANT-t: AP: *ARS: *AUR: Bell: CAPS:
CHAM: CON: *DROS: DUL: EUPHOR: FER:
HYO: KALI-c: Lach: LYC: MENY: Merc: NAT-s:
PAL: PHO: PLAT: *PULS: *RHUS-t: RUMX:
*RUT: SAMB: SANG: SEP: STRO: SUL: TARX:
VERB:

LYING RELIEVES
*AM-m: Arn: BELL: *BRY: *CALC-c: CALC-p:
Cham: COLO: *FER: IGN: *MANG: *NAT-m:
*NUX-v: *PIC-ac: PULS: Rhus-t: Sep: Sil:
*SQUIL: Stan: SUL:

LYING ON ABDOMEN RELIEVES
*BELL: Calc-p: CHEL: Cina: *COLO: Elap: EUP-
pf: Lach: *MED: NIT-ac: Par: *PHO: *POD:
PSOR: PULS: SEP: STAN:

LYING ON RIGHT SIDE AGGRAVATES
ALU: AM-m: BENZ-ac: BOR: Caus: CHEL: Iris:
KALI-c: MAG-m: *MERC: NUX-v: Pho: Rumx:
SPO: Stan:

LYING ON LEFT SIDE AGGRAVATES
ACO: Am-c: AP: ARG-n: BAR-c: BRY: Cact:
CARB-a: COLCH: Ip: Lyc: Naj: NAT-c: NAT-m:
NAT-s: PAR: Petr: *PHO: *PULS: SEP: Sil: SUL:
THU:

LYING WITH HEAD LOW AGGRAVATES
Ant-t: ARG-m: *ARS: BELL: Caps: Chin: Colch:
Con: GEL: HEP: *KALI-n: Lach: (Phos: in chest
conditions) PULS: Samb: Sang: Spig: Spong:

LYING ON BACK RELIEVES
*ACO: *ANAC: Arg-n: Bar-c: *BRY: Cald:
*CALC-c: *CARB-a: Cina: Con: Fer: Ign: Ip:
*KALI-c: Kre: LYC: Merc-c: Merc: Nat-s: Par-q:
*PHO: Ph-ac: *PULS: RHUS-t: Rut: Seng: Sil:
*STAN: Stry: Sul: Thu:

SITTING AGGRAVATES
AGAR: AM-m: Ap: ARS: Asaf: *CAPS: *CON:
*CYC: *DUL: *EUPHOR: Fer: *LYC: Mag-m:
Mur-ac: NUX-v: PHO: *PLAT: *PULS: *RHUS-t:
RUT: *SEP: SUL: *VERB: ZN:

STANDING AGGRAVATES
Alo: Bry: *COCCL: *CON: *CYC: Fer-p: Ign:
*LIL-t: NAT-m: Nat-s: NUX-m: *PULS: Rhus-t:
SEL: *SEP: *SUL: VAL: TUB:

WORSE WALKING AND LYING – BETTER SITTING
GNAPH:

RESTLESS OR MOTIONLESS

RESTLESS
*ACO: ARG-n: AP: ARN: *ARS: Bapt: BELL:
Bism: CALC-c: CAUST: CHAM: Cimic: Cina:
CUP: EUP-pf: FER: FER-p: *HYO: LYC: MAG-p:
*MERC: NUX-v: PHO: *PYRO: *PULS: *RHUS-t:
*SEP: STAPH: Stram: SUL: *TARN: Zn: Vib:

MOTIONLESS
*BRY: Cad-s: Colch: Coccl: Con: *GEL: Hell:
NUX-m: Phos:
(Compare "Inactive").

Note: BRY: is sometimes restless in spite of the pain any
movement may cause. There is no temporary
relief by moving as in BAP: RHUS-t: and PYRO:

SENSATIONS

BALL OR LUMP SENSATION
ARN: ASF: Aur: BRY: Cham: Chin: Cob: Gel:
*IGN: Kali-c: Kali-m: Lac-c: *LACH: Lil-t: LYC:
Merc-d: MERC-i-r: Mos: Nat-m: Nat-p: Nat-s: Nit-ac:
Nux-m: NUX-v: Paris: Pho: *PHYT: Plan: *PULS:
Raph: Rhus-t: Rumx: SABAD: Senec: *SEP: Spi:
Sul: VAL: Zn:

BURNING SENSATION
ACON: AGAR: ALL-c: *AP: *ARS: Bell: Bry:
CALAD: *CANTH: CAPS: Carb-a: Carb-v:
*CAUST: Cham: EQUIS: FER-p: Graph: Kre:
NAT-m: Ph-ac: *PHO: Pip-m: Rhus-t: SANG: Sec:
Staph: *SUL: Tar-h: etc.,

COLDNESS AND COLLAPSE
ARS: *CAMP: *CARB-v: VER-a:

PLUG, NAIL, WEDGE SENSATION
Agar, *ALOE: ANAC: Arn: Asaf: COFF: HEP:
*IGN: Lith: Mos: *NUX-v: PLAT: RAN-s: Rut:
*SPO: Sul: SUL-ac: *THU:

DRYNESS GENERAL
Aco: ALU: ARS: *BELL: BRY: Cald: Cam: Grap:
Held: Iod: Lach: Lyc: Mali: NAT-m: Nat-s: *NUX-m:
*NUX-v: Pho: Plb: PULS: RHUS-t: Sang: Sanic:
Sec-c: Sul: Tub:

DRYNESS PARTIAL
Aco: Alu: *BELL: Bry: Fer: Graph: Kali-bi: LYC:
NAT-m: *NUX-m: PHO: *PULS: Rhus-t: Sul:
Ver-a:

FAINT
ACO: *ARS: BRY: *CAUST: CARB-v: CHAM:
CHIN: CROT-h: DIG: *GLON: HEP: IGN: IOD:
*LACH: MOS: NUX-m: *NUX-v: OP: *PULS:
*SEP: SUL: VER-a: etc.,

FAINTNESS AFTER DIARRHOEA
ARS: NUX-v: VER-a:

FAINTNESS IN CROWDED CLOSE ROOM
AM-c: LYC: NAT-m: PHO: PLB: *PULS: SEP:

FAINTNESS AFTER COITION
AGAR: Dig: Nat-p: Sep:

FAINTNESS (WOMEN) DURING COITION
Murx: Orig: PLAT:

FAINTNESS DURING MENSES
Lach: NUX-m: Nux-v: Sep:

FAINTNESS ON RISING UP
*BRY: Merc-i-f: *PHYT: VER-v: Vib:

FAINTNESS KNEELING
SEP:

FAINTNESS AT SIGHT OF BLOOD
NUX-v:

FAINTNESS FROM EMOTIONAL UPSET
IGN:

HARD-BED SENSATION
*ARN: *BAP: Con: Dro: FER-p: Gel: Kali-c: Nux-v: Pho: Plat: *PYRO: RHUS-t: SIL: TIL:

NAUSEA
*AETH: *ANT-c: *ANT-t: *ARS: Bap: BELL: BIS: *BRY: Carb-v: Cham: *COCCL: *CAD-s: Colch: Cup: Dig: Dul: EUP-pf: *GEL: HEP: Ign: *IP: IRIS: Kali-bi: Lyc: Nat-m: Nit-ac: *NUX-v: PETR: Pho: Pilo: PULS: *PYRO: Rhus-t: Rob: Sang: Sep: Sil: Sul: TAB: *VER-a:

NUMBNESS
*ACO: AGAR: Ap: Ars: BERB: CALC-p: CAMP: Carb-v: Caus: Cham: *COCCL: CON: GEL: GLO: *GRAP: Kali-c: *LYC: Nux-m: Nux-v: OP: PHO: Ph-ac: PLAT: Plb: *PULS: *RHUS-t: SEC-c: STRAM: Thu: Zn:

PART LAME OR NUMB
CHIN: *PULS: *RHUS-t:

30

SINKING SENSATION
Alu: BRY: Dul: GLO: Kali-c: LACH: Lyc: NAT-m:
PHO: Rhus-t: Tab:

FALLING SENSATION
Bell: Thu:

SINKING THROUGH FLOOR
Hyo: Pho:

SINKING THROUGH BED
Bry: (Compare "Vertigo").

BED SWAYING UP AND DOWN
BELL:

SPLINTER SENSATION, PRICKING
*AESC: AGAR: Alu: All-c: Ap: *ARG-n: ARS:
Bry: Caps: Collin: *HEP: KALI-bi: KALI-c: Merc-i-fl:
Nat-m: Nat-p: *NIT-ac: Paeo: Pho: Rat: Rhus-t:
Sabad: *SIL: Sul: Symp: Thu: Val: Ver-a:

TINGLING OR ITCHING
*ACO: AGAR: Alu: Ant-t: Ap: Ars: CALC-c:
Carb-s: Carb-v: *CAUS: Chel: Grap: LYC: Mag-c:
MERC: Mez: Nat-m: Pho: PSO: PULS: RHUS-t:
Sep: SIL: Spo: STAP: *SUL: Sul-io: Urt-u:

TIGHT BAND
Alu: Anac: Ap: Arg-n: Ars: *BELL: *CACT: Caps:
Carb-v: Chel: Chin: *CIMI: *COCCL: Colo: Con:
*GRAP: IGN: LACH: Lyc: Mag-p: *MERC: Nat-m:
*NIT-ac: *NUX-v: Pho: PLAT: PLB: PULS:
RHUS-t: SELE: SIL: *STAN: SUL:

TREMBLING
Agar: *ANT-t: *ARG-n: *ARS: CALC-c: Chel:
*CIMI: *COCCL: *GEL: Grap: IOD: Ipec:
*LACH: *MERC: *NUX-v: *OP: *PULS: *RHUS-t:
Samb: Sil: STAP: Stro: *SUL: Sul-ac: Ver-a: ZN:

NERVOUS SHUDDERING
Aco: *ARN: *ARS: BELL: Cham: CIMI: Cina:
*GEL: Glo: Hyp: Ign: LED: NAT-m: *NUX-v:
PULS: RHUS-t: Sep: SIL: SPI: Thu: Zn:

SENSITIVITY

IN GENERAL
ACO: *ARG-n: Arn: Ars: Aur: *BELL: CHAM:
*CHIN: COFF: FER-p: GEL: *HEP: *IGN:
*LACH: *LYC: *NAT-m: *NIT-ac: *NUX-v:
*PHO: *PULS: SEP: *SIL: *SUL: *VAL:

SENSITIVE TO DRAUGHTS
ACO: Ars: *BELL: *CALC-c: *CALC-p: CAPS:
CHAM: *CHIN: *HEP: *KALI-c: LACH: LYC:
MERC: *NUX-v: PHO: PH-ac: PHYT: RHOD:
*RHUS-t: SEP: *SIL: Squil: *SUL:

LIGHT AGGRAVATES
*ACON: *ARS: *BELL: BRY: *CALC-c: *CHIN:
Colch: Con: *EUPHR: EUP-pf: *GEL: GLO:
*GRAP: HEP: Kali-bi: KALI-p: Lac-c: Lach:
*LYC: Lys: Mag-p: MERC-c: *MERC: Nat-c:
*NAT-s: *NAT-m: Nux-m: *NUX-v: *PHO:
*RHUS-t: *SEP: SIL: STRA: *SUL:

SENSITIVE TO MUSIC
ACON: AMBR: CHAM: DIG: GRAP: KRE:
LYC: *NAT-c: NAT-m: *NAT-s: *NUX-v: PHO:
PH-ac: SABI: *SEP: TAR:

SENSITIVE TO NOISE
*ACO: ARN: ASAR: *BELL: *BOR: BRY:
*CHIN: CON: *FER-p: *GEL: HEP: Ign: Kali-bi:
*KALI-c: *KALI-p: LACH: LYC: Mag-m: MERC:
NAT-m: Nat-s: *NIT-ac: *NUX-v: *OP: PHO:
PULS: *SEP: *SIL: *THER: *ZN:

SENSITIVE TO ODOURS
Ars: Aur: BELL: COCCL: Doff: *COLCH: Eup-pf:
Grap: Ign: Ip: LACH: Lyc: MERC-i-f: Nux-m:
*NUX-v: SABAD: Sang: *SEP: Stan: Sul: Ther: Thu:

SENSITIVITY TO TOUCH
See "Pressure and Touch".

SENSITIVE TO A JAR OR STEPPING HARD

ACON: *ARN: ARS: *BELL: Berb: *BRY: CHIN: *CIC: COCCL: *CON: Fer-p: GLO: GRAP: HAM: HEP: *HYP: *LACH: LIL-t: NAT-m: *NIT-ac: NUX-v: PHO: PULS: *RHUS-t: *SEP: *SIL: SPI: SUL: *THER: THU:

SENSITIVE TO SLIGHTEST NOISE ON GOING TO SLEEP

CALC-c:

HEAD SENSITIVE TO COLD AIR

Caus: Chin: Hep: Nux-v: Sil: AT NIGHT Pho:

SIDES IN GENERAL

ALTERNATING

Abro: Agar: Alo: AMB: Ant-c: Ap: Arn: ARS: Ben-ac: Bell: Berb: Cam: CAN: CIMI: COCCL: Colo: Croc: Cup: Fer-p: Glo: IGN: Iris: Kali-c: *LAC-c: Lach: *LYC: Nat-p: Parf: *PHO: Poly: PSO: PULS: Sep: Strop: *SUL: Sul-ac: Tab: Tarn: Val: Xan: Zn:

LEFT SIDE

ACON: ANT-c: ANT-t: APIS: ARG-n: *ASAF: ASAR: Ast-r: Calc-f: CAPS: CINA: CLEM: CROC: EUPHO: GRAP: KALI-c: KRE: *LACH: Lil-t: Mag-s: MERC-i-r: MEZ: Nat-s: OLD: Par-q: *PHO: RHUS-t: Sabad: SELE: *SEP: Sil: Spig: SQUIL: Stan: *SUL: Thu:

LEFT GOING TO RIGHT

Ars: Brom: Calc-c: Cap: All-c: Fer: Ip: *LACH: *MERC-i-r: Nux-m: Puls: RHUS-t: Sabad: Stan: Tarx:

RIGHT SIDE

AP: ARG-n: ARS: AUR: BAP: *BELL: BOR: BRY: *CALC-c: CANTH: Caus: *CHEL: COLO: CON: CROT-h: FER-p: Gel: Hep; Iris: Kalm: *LYC: LYS: MERC: MERC-i-fl: Naj: NIT-ac: NUX-v: PULS: RAN-b: RAN-s: RAT: Rumx: SABAD: Sang: SARS: SIL: STAPH: Sul-ac: TARN:

RIGHT GOING TO LEFT
Aco: Amb: Am-c: AP: BELL: Calc-p: CAUS: Chel:
Cup: LIL-t: *LYC: *MERC-i-fl: PHO: Rumx:
SABAD: Sang: Sul-ac: VER-a:

LOWER RIGHT ABDOMEN (APPENDIX)
LACH: in High Potency (Compare "Vomiting").
Call a Doctor at once.

Note: For particular sides see under "Headache" for
head, under "Chest" for lungs and under
"Throat and Larynx" for throat etc.

SLEEPY OR WAKEFUL

SLEEPINESS — DROWSINESS
AETH: ALU: ANT-c: *ANT-t: AP: ARS: *BAP:
*BELL: Calc-c: CARB-v: CAUS: *CHEL: CHIN:
CLEM: CROC: Echi: FER-p: *GEL: GRAP:
KALI-a: *LACH: *MERC-c: *NUX-m: *NUX-v:
*OP: PHO: *PH-ac: PIC-ac: Pip-m: PODO: PULS:
SUL: THU:

SLEEPINESS BY DAY YET SLEEPLESS AT NIGHT
Fer: Mos: Op: Ph-ac: PULS: Rhus-t: SUL:

FLOW OF SALIVA DURING SLEEP
Lach: *MERC: PHO: Rhus-t:

RESTLESS AND TOSSING ABOUT
*ACO: *ARS: BAR-c: *BELL: CHAM: CHIN.
IOD: *LYC: *PULS: *PYRO: *RHUS-t: *SIL
*SUL: THU: etc.

SLEEPLESSNESS
Aco: Arg-n: *ARS: BELL: Bels: BRY: Cad-s
CACT: CALC-c: CHAM: Chin: COCCL: *COFF
Cycl: HEP: *HYO: Kali-a: Kali-c: *KALI-p: LACH
MERC-c: MERC: *NUX-v: OP: PHO: PLB: *PULS
RHUS-t: SEP: SIL: STAN: STAP: *SUL: THU:

SLEEPLESS FROM FLOW OF IDEAS – ACTIVE MIND
   *ARS: *CALC-c: *COFF: Gel: *HEP: Hyo: Ign:
   KALI-c: LACH: LYC: NAT-m: *NUX-v: Op:
   *PULS: PYROG: SEP: SIL: STAP: SUL:

SLEEPLESS ALTHOUGH SLEEPY
   Ap: BELL: Cham: Chel: Hep: Kali-p: Op: Pho: Pul:
   Sep: etc.

SLEEPLESS ON ONCE WAKING
   Ars: Lach: NAT-m: Sil: Sul:

SLEEPLESS FROM GRIEF
   Ign: Kali-br: NAT-m:

DREAMS OF FALLING
   THU:

WORSE AFTER SLEEP
   Ap: Ars: Bell: Chin: Hep: *LACH: LYC: NUX-v:
   Op: Pho: Puls: Rhus-t: SPO: Stram: SUL:

SLEEP AMELIORATES
   Ars: COCCL: Cof: Colch: Merc: NUX-v: Pall:
   PHO: Pul: Sang: Sep: Zinc:

THIRST OR THIRSTLESS

THIRST INCREASED
*ACO: Ant-c: *ARS: BELL: *BISM: *BRY:
CALC-c: CALC-s: CAPS: CAUS: *CHAM: *CHIN:
Cina: DIG: *EUP-pf: *FER-p: HEP: IOD: LYC:
MERC-c: *MERC: *NAT-m: NAT-s: Nux-v: Op:
*PHO: Pyro: *RHUS-t: Sec-c: SEP: SIL: *STRAM:
*SUL: Tarn: *VER-a: VER-v:

THIRST FOR LITTLE AND OFTEN
Aco: Ant-t: Ap: *ARS: Bell: Carb-v: *CHIN:
COLOC: *LYC: Nat-a: Pyro: Rhus-t: SUL: Vera-a:

THIRST FOR MUCH AT A TIME
Ars: *BRY: CHIN: *EUP-pf: FER-p: Lil-t: *NAT-m:
*PHO: Podo: *SUL: *VER-a:

THIRST FOR MUCH AT LONG INTERVALS
*BRY: Podo: SUL: Ver-a:

THIRSTLESS DURING FEVER
Aesc: Aeth: Ant-t: *AP: CARB-v: CINA: FER:
*GEL: Hell: IGN: *IP: NUX-m: NIT-ac: *PULS:
SABAD: SEP: SUL:

THIRSTY BUT DOES NOT DRINK
Bell: Hyos: Lach:

THIRSTY FOR SMALL QUANTITIES INFREQUENTLY
*ARS: BAPT: CHIN: Hell: Lac-c: LACH: *LYC
Merc-i-r: Pyro: RHUS-t: SUL:
Ant-t: and Ip: both have variable thirst.

TIMES

(Greenwich Mean Times)
(Deduct one hour for Summer Time)

EARLY MORNING AGGRAVATION (4 a.m. – 9 a.m.)
Agar: *AM-m: *ANT-t: Arg-m: Ars-io: *AUR: Bor:
Bov: BRY: *CALC-c: Calc-p: Cann-s: Carb-an:
CARB-v: Cham: *CHEL: Cina: Con: CROC: Echi:
Elap: FERR-p: Hep: KALI-bi: Kali-c: Kali-n:
*LACH: Naj: *NAT-m: NAT-s: NIT-ac: *NUX-v:
Onos: Petr: *PHO: Ph-ac: PODO: Puls: RHOD:
*RHUS-t: Rumx: Sabad: Sep: *SCIL: *SUL: Val:
Verb:

6 a.m.
Alo: ALU: Arn: Bov: Fer: HEP: Lyc: NUX-v: Sil:
Sul: *VER-a:

7 a.m.
*EUP-pf: HEP: Nat-c: NUX-v: *POD: Sep:

8 a.m.
*EUP-pf: NUX-v:

8 a.m. – 12 noon
Arg: Cact: Can: Chin: CHIN-s: EUP-pf: GEL: Nat-c:
*NAT-m: Nux-v: Pho: Pod: Sabad: Sep: Stan: SUL:
Sul-ac:

9 a.m.
Bry: Cedr: *CHAM: *EUP-pf: KALI-bi: Kali-c:
Lac-c: Nat-m: Nux-v: Sep: Sul-ac: VERB:

9 a.m. – 12 noon
Arg-m: *CANN-s: Carb-v: Guaiac: Hep: Laur:
*NAT-c: NAT-m: Nux-m: Pod: Ran-b: Rhus-t:
*SABA: *SEP: Sil: *STAN: *SUL: Sul-ac: Val: Vio-t:

8 a.m. – 2 p.m.
CHIN:

10 a.m.
ARS: Bor: Chin: EUP-pf: *GEL: IOD: NAT-c:

*NAT-m: Petr: PHO: RHUS-t: Sep: Sil: STAN: SUL: Thu:

10 a.m. – 3 p.m.
Chin-s: Nat-m: Tub:

11 a.m.
Ars: Bap: Cact: CHIN-s: Coccl: GEL: Hyds: Hyo: Indm: IP: LACH: Mag-p: Nat-c: *NAT-m: Nat-p: NUX-v: PHO: Puls: RHUS-t: Sep: Stan: *SUL: ZN:

12 noon
Ant-c: *ARG-m: Chel: Chin: Elap: EUP-pf: Kali-c: Lach: NAT-m: Nux-m: NUX-v: Pho: *POLYP: SIL: Spig: Stram: SUL: Val: Verb:

AFTERNOON (12 noon – 6 p.m.)
Agar: Alo: *ALU: Amb: *ANG: Ant-c: *AP: Asaf: *BELL: Bry: Chel: *CHIN: CIMIC: Colch: Colo: DIG: Hell: IGN: KALI-n: *LYC: *PULS: *RHUS-t: *SEP: *SIL: SUL: THU: *ZN:

1 p.m.
ARS: Cact: Chel: Cina: Grat: Kali-c: LACH: Mag-c: Pho: PULS:

2 p.m.
Ars: Chel: EUP-pf: Fer: Gel: LACH: Mag-p: Nit-ac: PULS: Rhus-t:

3 p.m.
Ang: Ant-t: AP: ARS: Asaf: *BELL: Ced: Chel: CHI-s: Con: Nat-m: Samb: Sang: STAP: THU:

3 p.m. – 7 p.m.
Indm: Phos: PULS: *SEP: SIL:

4 p.m.
AESC: ANAC: AP: Ars: Cact: *CAUS: CED: *CHEL: CHI-s: *COLO: GEL: Hyo: Hep: Ip: *LYC: MANG: NAT-m: Nat-s: Nit-ac: NUX-v: PULS: Rhus-t: Sul: Verb:

4 p.m. – 8 p.m.
AP: CAUS: Chel: Colo: Dig: FER-p: Hell: Hyo:

*LYC: Nit-ac: Nux-m: Pho: Plat: PULS: RHUS-t: Sabad: Sep: SUL: Zn:

5 p.m.
Alu: Caus: CED: CHIN: *COLO: Con: *GEL: *HEP: Hypr: KALI-c: LYC: Nat-m: NUX-v: PULS: RHUS-t: Sul: *THU: Tub: Val:

EVENING (6 p.m. – 9 p.m.)
*ACO: All-c: Amb: AM-c: Ant-c: ANT-t: ARG-n: ARN: *BELL: BRY: CAPS: CAUS: Chel: Colch: *CYC: *EUPHR: Flu-ac: Hell: Hyo: *KALI-n: Kali-s: *LYC: Mag-c: *MENY: MERC: Mez: *NIT-ac: PHO: *PLAT: Plb: *PULS: *RAN-sc: Rumx: Sep: Stan: STRO: *SUL: Sul-ac: Val: Zn:

6 p.m.
Ant-t: CED: *HEP: Kali-c: Nat-m: *NUX-v: Petr: *PULS: RHUS-t: SEP: SIL:

7 p.m.
Alu: Bov: CED: Chi-s: Fer: Gamb: Gel: *HEP: Ip: *LYC: Nat-m: NAT-s: NUX-v: Petr: Puls: Pyro: RHUS-t: SEP: Sul: Tarn:

8 p.m.
Alu: BOV: Caus: Coff: Elap: Hep: Mag-c: *MERC-i-r: Merc: Pho: RHUS-t: *SUL:

8 p.m. – Midnight
Arg-n: BOV: *BRY: Carb-v: Gel: Lyc: Mur-ac: Pho: Puls: Rumx: Stan: Sul:

NIGHT (9 p.m. – 4 a.m.)
*ACO: ARN: *ARS: Bell: *CHAM: CHIN: Cimic: Coff: *COLCH: Con: Dulc: *FER: *GRAP: *HEP: Hyo: Iod: Jal: Kali-c: KALI-io: MAG-c: Mag-m: Mang: Mep: *MERC: *NIT-ac: Pho: *PLB: PSOR: Puls: Rhus-t: SIL: STRO: SUL: *SYPH: *ZN:

9 p.m.
Ars: BOV: *BRY: GEL: Merc:

10 p.m.
Ars: Bov: Cham: *CHI-s: GRAP: Ign: Lach: Petr:

Podo: Puls:

11 p.m.
Aral: Ars: Bell: *CACT: Calc-c: Carb-an: RUMX: Sul:

12 Midnight
*ACO: ARG-n: *ARS: Calc-c: Calad: Canth: CAUS: CHIN: Dig: DROS: FER: Kali-c: Lach: Lyc: MAG-m: MERC: Mur-ac: Nat-m: Nux-m: NUX-v: Op: PHO: Puls: RHUS-t: Samb: Stram: Sul: Ver-a:

1 a.m.
*ARS: Carb-v: Chin: Mag-m: PULS:

2 a.m.
*ARS: BENZ-ac: Canth: CAUS: Dros: Fer: Graph: HEP: Iris: *KALI-bi: *KALI-c: Kali-p: Lach: Lachn: Lyc: Mag-c: Mez: Nat-m: Nat-s: NIT-ac: Ptel: PULS: Rumx: Sars: SIL: Spig: Sul:

3 a.m.
AM-c: AM-m: Ant-t: ARS: *BRY: Calc-c: Canth: CED: Chin: Fer: Iris: *KALI-c: MAG-c: NAT-m: NUX-v: Podo: PSOR: RHUS-t: Samb: Sele: Sep: Sil: *SUL: THU:

4 a.m.
ALU: AM-m: Anac: AP: ARN: BOR: CAUS: *CED: Chel: Colo: CON: Fer: IGN: Kali-c: *LYC: MUR-ac: NAT-s: Nit-ac: *NUX-v: *PODO: PULS: Sep: Sil: Stan: Sul: Ver-a:

4 a.m. – 8 a.m.
Alu: Arn: Aur: Bry: Chel: EUP-pf: *FER-p: Hep: Kali-bi: Lach: NAT-m: Nux-v: *PODO: Rumx: SUL: Ver-a:

5 a.m.
Alo: AP: *CHIN: Dros: FER-p: KALI-c: Kali-io: NAT-m: Nat-p: Ph-ac: PODO: Rumx: Sep: Sil: *SUL:

6 a.m. – Noon
ARS:

VERTIGO

VERTIGO IN GENERAL
Ars: ACO: Ail: Ap: Arg-m: Bap: *BELL: *BRY:
CALC-c: Calc-s: Carb-v: *CHEL: *COCCL: *CON:
Cup: Cyc: Dig: Dul: *EUP-pf: Fer: *GEL: Kali-bi:
LYC: NAT-m: *NUX-v: Op: Petr: *PHO: *PULS:
RHUS-t: Sang: Sec-c: Sep: Sil: Sul: TAB: Ver-a:

THE ACT OF SITTING UP IN BED OR RISING FROM A CHAIR
ACON: *BRY: *CHEL: *COCCL: Kali-bi: Kali-p:
Merc-i-f: NAT-s: NUX-v: Pho: Phyt: Puls: RHUS-t:
Sil: Sul: Ver-v: Vib:

AS IF INTOXICATED
*CHEL: *COCCL: EUP-pf: *GEL: *NUX-v:
*PULS: Lyc:

FLOATING SENSATION
Hyper: Lac-c: Lach: Manc: Mez: Nux-m: Sep: Valer:

REELING – STAGGERING
AGAR: ALUM: Arg-n: ARS: Bell: Caps: CAUST:
*CHEL: GEL: LYC: NUX-m: *NUX-v: *PHO:
*PYRO: *RHUS-t: Sec-c: Stram:

SINKING THROUGH THE BED
*BRY: Calc-p: Chin: Lach: Lyc: Rhus-t:

THE ACT OF LYING DOWN
Bell:

OBJECTS APPEAR TO BE MOVING TO THE RIGHT
NAT-sal:

STOOPING AGGRAVATES
*ACON: Bar-c: Bell: Bry: Glo: Iod: *KALM: Nux-v:
*PULS: *SUL: Ther:

TURNING IN BED OR MOVING THE HEAD WHILE LYING
*BELL: *BRY: Calc-c: *CON: Gel: Pho:

WORSE ASCENDING
  *CALC-c: Sul:

WORSE CLOSING THE EYES
  Arn: Chel: LACH: Mag-p: Nat-m: Sep: Ther: Thu:

CLOSING THE EYES RELIEVES
  *CON: *GELS:

WORSE DESCENDING
  *BOR: Con: Gel: Plat: SANIC:

VERTIGO BEFORE VOMITING
  Nat-s:

VERTIGO WITH VOMITING
  *ARS: *CHEL: BRY: Glon: GEL: Lach: Merc:
  *NAT-s: NUX-v: Puls: Sang: *VER-a: Sul:

VISION AFFECTED
  *CYC: *FER: *GEL: *NUX-v: Strop:

WHEN RISING:
  ACON: *BRY: Chel: *FER: Coccl: Kali-p: Merc-i-f:
  NAT-m: Nux-v: PHO: Phyt: RHUS-t: TAB:

WHEN LOOKING UP
  Calc-c: Chin-ar: *GRANAT: *KALI-p: Petrol:
  *PULS: *SIL: Tab: Thu:

WHIRLING, TURNING IN A CIRCLE
  BELL, *BRY: *CHEL: *CON: Cycl: Lyc: Nux-v:
  *PULS: Rhus-t: Sabad:

NAUSEA
  See under "Sensations".

CHEST

Bronchitis, Broncho-pneumonia, Pneumonia, Pleurisy, Pleuro-pneumonia.
Use 30 Potency or higher.

VERY EARLY STAGE
*ACO: BAP: *BELL: *FER-p: GEL: *IP: Merc: Nit-ac: Op: Pyro:

DEVELOPED STAGE
*BRY: Caps: *CHEL: *KALI-c: Kali-bi: LACH: Lob: LYC: *NAT-s: *PHO: PULS: Ran-b: Rhus-t: Sang: SENEG: VER-v:

Note: VER-v: can cause cardiac depression.

LATER STAGE
*ANT-t: AMM-c: Arn: Carb-an: CARB-v: Canth: Kre: TERB: *SUL:

SIDES
Either Side, ANT-t: PHO:

Left. ACON: (Bell: rarely). (Bry: rarely). KALI-c: LACH: NAT-s: PHO: Ran-b: SUL:

Left Apex. ACON: LACH:

Left lower lobe. KALI-c: NAT-s: Rumx:

Pain through to left shoulder blade. SUL:

Right. ARS: BELL: BRY: CHEL: FER-p: Kali-c: LYC: MERC: Sul:

Right lower lobe. CHEL: KALI-c: MERC: PHO:

Note: Ars: is rarely required in a case of collapse, then it must be followed quickly after its reaction by another remedy often either Phos: or Sul:

Pain goes under arm to back. BRY:

Right lower lobe extending to back. MERC:

Right lower lobe extending to right shoulder blade:
   CHEL:

RELIEVED
   Lying with head back. ANT-t:

   Lying on painful side. BRY:

   Movement. SENEG:

   Propped up on back with arms raised from sides or above head. PULS:

   Propped up with no constriction or weight of bed-clothes. ANT-t:

   Propped up with no constriction on neck or chest and desire for air to be fanned. CARB-v:

   Propped up with head back and chin up. PHO:

   Propped up firmly to avoid movement. BRY:

   Sitting up and leaning forward. CHEL: KALI-c:

   Sitting up with elbows on knees. KALI-c:

COUGH RELIEVED BY
   Current of fresh air. BRY: IP:

   Holding chest: BRY:

   Sitting up and holding chest: NAT-s:

   Sitting up with head tilted well back. HEP:

WORSE
   Motion. *BRY: CHEL: FER-p: KALI-c:

   Lying on affected side. ACON: BELL: HEP: PULS:

PAIN
   Aching chest wall. ANT-t: NAT-s: PULS: PYRO: SENEG:

   Stabbing: ACON: early. *BRY: CHEL: HEP: *KALI-c: LACH: MERC: NAT-s:

44

Notes: AMM-c: and ANT-t: are very similar but AMM-c: is worse for cold and ANT-t: is worse for heat.

DOSAGE
Use one tablet of the 30 potency every two hours for the first three doses. Then continue every four hours. After the temperature is normal in the evening, it is advisable to give a further three doses at four-hourly intervals.

FOR INFANTS
IP: is of particular use for young people when symptoms agree, i.e. coarse rattling in the chest, nausea or vomiting – generally clean tongue and no thirst, respiration or wheezing – the 6 potency generally.

Both Bry: and Nat-s: have pain in the chest when coughing – that of Bry: is dry and Nat-s: is loose.

DIARRHOEA

FROM ANGER. CHAM: *COLOC: NUX-v: STAPH:

FROM BAD FOOD. *ARS: (Compare under "Cause").

WHEN BABY IS TEETHING. CHAM:

FROM BAD NEWS. GELS:

FROM COLD BATHING. ANT-c: POD:

FROM EXPOSURE TO COLD WIND. *ACO:

FROM GETTING WET. ACO: CALC-c: *DULC: *RHUS-t:

FROM 'NERVES' OR FRIGHT OR ANTICIPATION
ACO: *ARG-n: CHAM: Coff: *GEL: Hyo: Ign: OP: PH-ac: Pod: PULS: VER-a:

PAINFUL
Ars: Bry: Cham: *COLOC: Merc: Merc-c: POD: Rhe: *RHUS-t: Sul: etc.

PAINLESS (sometimes)
ARS: Calc-s: *CHIN: FER: Hyo: Lyc: NAT-s: PHO: *PH-ac: *POD: Puls: Pyro: Stam: Sul: VER-a:

PROSTRATING
ANT-t: *ARS: *CAMP: *VER-a:

NOT PROSTRATING
AP: Ph-ac:

SCANTY BUT FREQUENT
ARS: MERC-c: NUX-v:

WITH SHARP COLICKY PAINS RELIEVED BY HARD PRESSURE AND BENDING DOUBLE
*COLOC: *MAG-p: RHUS-t:

WITH VOMITING. See "Vomiting".

DIARRHOEA FROM BEER. KALI-bi:

FAINTNESS AFTER DIARRHOEA. See "Sensations".

DIARRHOEA ONLY AT NIGHT. Chin:

DIARRHOEA ONLY DAYTIME. Petr:

DIARRHOEA CAUSED BY ANTIBIOTICS: NIT-ac:30.

EARS

IN GENERAL
Acon: Aur: *BELL: CALC-c: Cham: *FER-p: Grap: HEP: Hyd: Lyc: Mang: *MERC: Petr: Pho: Pic-ac: Plant: PSOR: *PULS: *SIL: SUI: TELL:

ACHING
ACON: *BELL: *CHAM: *FER-p: NUX-v: *PULS:

DISCHARGING
*CALC-c: Con: HEP: LYC: *MERC: Pho *PULS: Sil: Vio-o:

INNER EAR INFLAMED
*FER-p: *MERC-s: Pho: Sul: Tell:

STOPPED OR BLOCKED FEELING
Ars: Con: *KALI-m: Lyc: Merc: *PULS: Sil:

THROAT EXTENDING TO EARS
(See under "Throat").

TUBES – EUSTACHIAN
Bar-m: Calc-c: Grap: Hyds: *KALI-m: Kali-s:
MERC-d: Nux-v: Petr: Puls: Sang: Sil:

EARACHE ASSOCIATED WITH TOOTHACHE
CHAM: PLANT: SIL:

MIDDLE EAR
Aur: *CAPS: Hep: MERC: Sil: *SYMP:
(use 1 part tincture with 2 parts sterile water in ear
three times a day.)

WAX CAUSING PAIN
Insert 3 drops of Mullein Oil in the ear.

WORSE WARMTH OF BED
*MERC: Nux-v:

BETTER WRAPPING UP
Cham: Dulc: *HEP: Mag-p: Sep:

EYES

IN GENERAL
Aco: AGAR: ALL-c: Ap: ARG-n: ARS: *BELL:
Bry: *CALC-c: CALC-io: Caus: *EUPHR: FER-p:
*GEL: Grap: HEP: LYC: *MERC: MERC-c:
NAT-m: Nux-v: Pho: Phys: *PULS: RHUS-t: RUT:
Sep: *SUL: *SYMP: Ver-a: Vio-o: Zn:

CONJUNCTIVITIS
ACO: Ap: *ARG-n: Ars: BELL: ALL-c: *EUPHR:
*FER-p: Kali-bi: Merc: *PULS: Rhus-t: SUL:

EYEBALLS, SORE
Arn: Bap: Bell: BRY: Chel: *CIMIC: *EUP-pf:
*GEL: LACH: Merc: Pho: PHYT: Podo: Rhus-t:
Sang: Sep: Ther:

EYELIDS, TARSI
Bov: Fer-p: Merc: *PULS: Stap: SUL: Val:

EYELIDS, STYES
Calc-fl: Fer-p: Grap: PULS: STAP: Sul: Zn:

LACHRYMATION (WATERING EYES)
Ars: BELL: CALC-c: *ALL-c: Colch: *EUPHR:
Flu-ac: Ip: Kali-p: Kre: MERC: *NAT-m: Nit-ac:
Op: Pho: *PULS: RHUS-t: *RUT: Sabad: Sil:
*STAP: Stram: *SUL:

CYSTS ON EYELID
CALC-fl: 3x

EYE-STRAIN
*RUT: NAT-m: Seneg:

EYES WATERING DURING COLDS
*ALL-c: Ars: *CARB-v: *EUPHR: Gels: Kali-io:
Nat-m: *NUX-v: Phos: Phyt: Puls: Sabad: Tell:

EYES WATERING WITH COUGHING
Eup-pf: *EUPHR: HEP: *NAT-m: Phyt: *PULS:
SABAD: Scil: *SQUIL:

EYES INJECTED (BLOODSHOT)
*ACO: AP: ARG-m: *ARN: *BELL: All-c: Glo:
Led: MERC: Nat-m: Nux-v:
(See also Part 1, "Facial Appearance".)

BLACK EYE
ARN: LED: *SYMP:

FOREIGN BODY IN EYE
*ACON: ARN: EUPHR: Hyp: SIL: *SYMP:

EYES BURN OR SMART
ACON: ALL-c: ALU: AP: *ARS: BELL: Bry:
Calc-c: Cham: Chin: *EUPHR: Grap: KALI-bi:
Kali-c: KALI-io: LACH: LYC: MERC: Merc-i-r:
Mez: *NAT-m: PULS: Pho: Phyt: RHUS-t: Ruta:
Sabad: Sep: *SUL:

FOR HAY FEVER
See under "Nose".

PUPILS ENLARGED OR CONTRACTED
See under "Facial Appearance".

DROOPING EYELIDS
See under "Facial Appearance".

EYES HURT WHEN COUGHING
Seneg:

NOSE AND ACCESSORY CAVITIES

IN GENERAL
Aco: Aesc: Alu: ARS: AUR: Calc-c: Grap: HEP:
*HYDS: Ign: Iod: *KALI-bi: KALI-io: KALI-m:
LYC: MERC: Merc-i-f: NAT-m: Nit-ac: Nux-v:
Pho: *PULS: Sabad: SEP: *SIL: Spi: SUL:

BLEEDING NOSE
*FER-p: FER-pic: SIL: *VIP:200.
Bovista very early morning during sleep.

EXTERNAL
AUR: Carb-v: Caus: Kali-c: MERC: Nat-c: Ph-ac:
Puls: RHUS-t: SEP: Spi: Sul:

ANTRUMS (SINUSES)
Ars: Cinnab: *HYDS: *KALI-bi: Kali-io: Lach:
Lyc: MERC: NAT-m: Pho: *SIL:6x

ACHING IN THE LIMBS AND FACE (From taking cold)
Acon: Bry: Dulc: *EUP-pf: *GELS: KALI-bi:
(Wandering pains) LACH: MERC: PYROG:
RHUS-t:
(See "Influenza").

COPIOUS WATERY DISCHARGE
Acon: *ALL-c: *ARS: Ars-io: Arum-t: Dulc:
*EUPHR: *GELS: Hep: Hyd: KALI-io: MERC:
Nat-ar: NAT-c: NAT-m: Quil: Sabad: Sang-n: THU:
(For Hay Fever see under "Eyes").

49

HILLINESS
Ars: Bry: Calc-c: *GELS: Ip: *NUX-v: Pho: Rhus-t:

Note "Stopped-up" nose dry. Nux-v:
"Stopped-up" nose sensation with watery discharge. Cham:

DISCHARGE ACRID
All-c: Ars: Gels: Kali-bi: Kali-iod: Merc: Nux-v: Sul:

SHIVERING AT START OF A COLD
BRY: EUP-pf: *GELS: IP: KALI-io: *NUX-v: *PYRO: RHUS-t:

SNEEZING IN GENERAL
*ALL-c: ARS: Ars-io: Bry: *CARB-v: CINA: Cocc: Eup-pf: GEL: Ign: Kali-io: Merc: NAT-m: *NUX-v: PULS: *RHUS-t: SABAD: Sang: Scil: Seneg: SIL: *SUL:

SNEEZING – VIOLENT BOUTS
*ARS: EUP-pf: Euphr: *GELS: IP: KALI-bi: KALI-io: MERC: *NAT-m: *NUX-v: PYRO: *RHUS-t: *SABAD:

WORSE AT NIGHT
CARB-v: RHUS-t:

WITH PAIN IN THE HEAD FROM SNEEZING OR COUGHING
Eup-pf: *BRY: NAT-m: PHO: RUMX:

WITH PAIN IN ABDOMEN FROM SNEEZING OR COUGHING
BRY: DROS:

NOT BETTER FROM SWEATING
HEP: *MERC:

TEARS ACRID: BURNING OR HOT
Ap: *ARS: *EUPHR: KALI-io: Merc-c: NAT-m: RHUS-t: Sul:

TEARS BLAND
    ALL-c: GELS: PULS:

Note GELS: has tears either burning or bland:

HOT OR ACRID DISCHARGE FROM THE NOSE
    ACON: *ALL-c: *ARS: Ars-io: GELS: KALI-io:
    MERC: Merc-c: Nux-v: Sul:

BLAND DISCHARGE FROM NOSE
    ACON: CALC-c: *EUPHR: GELS: IOD: NAT-m:
    Pho: *PULS: SEP: SIL: Stap: Sul:
Note ACON: and GELS: can have either acrid or bland
    discharge from nose.

GREENISH DISCHARGE
    Bry: Carb-v: *KALI-bi: *KALI-io: *MERC: Nit-ac:
    PHO: *PULS: Rhus-t: SEP:

BLOOD STREAKED
    PHO:

YELLOWISH-GREEN DISCHARGE
    Alum: Calc-s: HEP: *HYDR: *KALI-bi:
    (stringy) *MERC: NAT-s: PHO: *PULS: SEP: SIL:
    Ther: THU:

YELLOW DISCHARGE
    Aur: CALC-c: CALC-s: *HEP: *HYDR: *KALI-
    bi: *KALI-io: Lach: *LYC: Mag-m: Nat-s: Nat-m:
    NAT-p: *NIT-ac: PHO: *PULS: RUMX: *SEP: Sil:
    *SUL: Ther: THU: Tub:

BROWN DISCHARGE
    Kali-s:

BLOODY DISCHARGE
    *ALL-c: Alum: Ap: *ARS: Aur: *BELL: Calc-s:
    Carb-v: Caust: CHIN: *FER-p: *HEP: Hydr:
    *KALI-bi: *KALI-io: LACH: *MERC: NIT-ac:
    Nux-v: *PHO: Puls: Sil: Sul:

WITH THROAT AFFECTED
Carb-an: Calc-p: LACH: *MERC: *NIT-ac: *NUX-v: *PHO: PHYT: RHUS-t: etc.

Note See also under "Throat and Larynx".

EUSTACHIAN TUBES
Bar-m: *KALI-m: Nux-v: Petr:

RIGHT SIDE
HYDS:

LEFT SIDE
Sang:

CATARRH
Asar: Calc-c: Kali-s: Petr: *PULS: Sil:

ITCHING
Calc-c: Nux-v: Petr: SIL:

HAY FEVER
Mixed Pollen and Grasses 30.

One tablet twice a week for six weeks before pollen starts.

During high pollen count – one tablet morning and night.

INFLUENZA

Influenza viruses change so quickly that almost any remedy might be required. The only reliable method is as stated in the Introduction by taking the symptoms of each patient. However, a few remedies have proved very useful and are listed below with their main symptoms (compare "Nose and Accessory Cavities").

BELLADONNA (sudden onset) or **FERRUM-phos:** are also likely first remedies to be considered with Aconite.

ACONITE. If taken at the first sneeze Aconite will often prevent a cold or 'flu from developing but it is not so effective if not take in the first 24 hours – main symptoms are: *Sudden Onset* from exposure to cold, dry North East winds – running nose like clear warm water – fever – *Thirsty* – Sleeplessness – *Restless* and *Anxious* – frequent sneezing – throat inflamed – larynx sensitive to cold air. The first remedy to think of in Croup – eyes water – throbbing pulses.

GELSEMIUM. Slow onset – often in mild weather. Heavy eyed – wishes to be left alone – *Drowsy* – *Shivers Up and Down the Back* – shaky hands – sensitive to draughts – mouth dry – *Not Thirsty*. Headache in back of head going over to above one eye – or like a tight band round the head above the ears – back of neck sore and stiff – *General Soreness in the Muscles* – eyes sensitive to light – eyeballs sore – sense of pressure at root of nose – common cold symptoms with violent sneezing – clear water pours from nose – sometimes a nose bleed if blown too hard – a feeling of blockage in the ears – slight loss of voice – sometimes mild diarrhoea – copious urination relieves – *Limbs Feel Heavy* – pressing in frontal sinuses – trembling.

BAPTISIA. Rapid onset – gastric 'flu – face dusky red – puffy – eyes heavy – confused – *Difficult to Concentrate* – very dirty tongue – foul mouth – lips tend to crack – bed feels hard – restless tender all over

53

– heavy offensive sweat – throat dark red and painful
– cannot swallow solids – earache with sensation of
obstruction. More often right ear – sometimes
mastoid infection – *Thirsty. Vomiting Very Offensive,
Diarrhoea* and colic – acute pains in joints –
movement hurts – *Great Prostration* high
temperature – feels top of head will fly off.
(Cimicifuga and China also give this symptom.)
Virus pneumonia (compare "Chest").

Note Influenzium antidotes Baptisia.

ARS: has gastric influenza symptoms also – (see
Example 1 in the Introduction).

KALI, BICHROMICUM. Chilly, rheumatism like pains
that *Move From Place to Place,* relieved by warmth.
Worse at 2 or 3 a.m. and 6 – 8 a.m. Nasal discharge
yellowish and *Stringy.* Bridge of nose feels blocked
and hot – sneezing causes pain from nose to corner of
eye. *Tensions in Antrums* – headache on one side
worse by movement but better by pressure – relief by
hot applications. *Sometimes the Pain is in one Small
Spot.* Throat and uvula swollen, also tonsils. *Putting
Out the Tongue Causes Pain.* Sensation of a hair on
the palate – mucus in larynx – tightness in chest –
going sometimes to bronchitis – cough almost like
whooping cough with stringy mucus. Ears and
Eustachian tubes feel blocked – middle ear can
become involved also external ear becomes swollen –
gastric catarrh may develop with nausea and
vomiting. *The Back of the Neck Feels Chilly.* Hands
and soles of feel feel bruised on pressure – nose feels
dry. Saliva tastes salty. *Sensation of Choking on
Lying Down.* Scabs form inside nose. Air in nose is
hot. Glands of neck swollen.

BRYONIA. Dry heat – *Slow Onset* – irritable if disturbed.
Dislikes being questioned – depressed – anxiety
about his affairs – may think he is not at home when
delirious – difficult to please. *Movement is Painful*
but in spite of that they are sometimes restless – very
thirsty for large quantities at a time – likes a cool
room. Tongue thickly coated white and dry – lips dry

– throat dry and burning. Painful swallowing – *Cough Causes Pain in Head or Chest* – intense headache in forehead; throbbing – *Relieved by Firm Pressure* – scalp sometimes sensitive – eyeballs sore – heat or burning sensation in nose – vomiting – hoarseness or loss of voice – constipation – pneumonia sometimes follows with stabbing pains in chest – *Worse Slightest Movement.*

EUPATORIUM perfoliatum. Rapid onset – aching pains all over in all the bones particularly the shin bones – as if they were broken – *Very Scanty Sweat* – shivery and sensitive to draughts – headache worse on the part lain on – or headache with sensation of heat on top of head. Nose feels blocked but has fluent discharge and continuous sneezing – eyeballs sore – the eyes water – lids inflamed – scalp sensitive – *Sensitive to Any Smell* – *Very Thirsty* for cold drinks – throat dry. Heat in trachea – pain in chest muscles and back – violent cough hurts head and chest – although the pains can cause restlessness sometimes, often they are so severe the patient dare not move – vomiting of bile occasionally – wrists as if dislocated.

RHUS, TOXICODENDRON. Slow onset – pains in muscles – *Constantly Changing Position Gives Temporary Relief* – Chilly – *Sensitive to Cold Draughts,* which starts patient sneezing – anxious – depressed – tearful – high or moderate temperature – *Worse at Night* – disturbed sleep – profuse sweat – dry mouth and lips. Little sores on lower lip and corners of mouth. Tongue has red tip and is hot and dry. Teeth may become sensitive – dry burning throat worse empty swallowing – better solids than liquids. Violent sneezing worse at night – hoarseness – cough hurts larynx. Headache at back of head – *Staggers if he Stands Up.* Patient feels cold on the surface and burning inside. Not very thirsty – just sips. Aching in bones – *Very Restless* – scalp sensitive.

MERCURIUS. Greasy looking face – hot and restless – *Worse at Night,* rise of temperature and *Profuse Sweat which does not Relieve* – headache relieved by pressure – frontal sinuses and antrums also the ears and face can all be affected – *Very Sensitive to Draughts*. Thirsty *The Mouth is a Guiding Symptom* – the tongue looks *Wet, Flabby and Dirty with Increased Saliva*. The breath is offensive – throat is inflamed and swollen. The glands below the jawbone are enlarged – swallowing can cause pain in the ears – blowing the nose too hard can cause bleeding – larynx and trachea painful, worse by coughing. Hoarseness or loss of voice – eyes red and watering – burning – sensitive to light. Heat of fire makes eyes smart – nose runs, watery discharge that burns upper lip – violent sneezing – later greenish discharge with pain to antrums – ears become painful and throb, the whole head becomes very sensitive. General stiffness in neck, back and limbs – movement is painful. Hands shaky – impatient and anxious – desires an even room temperature – vomiting or nausea.

PYROGENIUM. Fairly high temperature – *Mentally Overactive* – very talkative – sleepless – very hot but sensitive to slightest draught. Sweat rather offensive – aching pains all over – *Very Restless*. Intense headache – *Throbbing,* relieved by pressure. Mouth dry – thirst for small quantities – tongue dry and brown – violent sneezing, worse from cold draught. Nose blocked first one side then the other. Larynx feels raw and burning. Cough with yellow mucus. Ringing in ears – they feel blocked, more often right ear. Frontal sinuses feel blocked – pressing pain above the eyes. *Intense Pulsations* sensative to light – taste putrid – no appetite – throat painful to swallow – diarrhoea with pains – *Fairly Low Temperature and Rapid Pulse or High Temperature and Slow Pulse*. Thumping heart. Vomiting after even a sip of water.

NUX VOMICA. Like Aconite from cold, dry winds – *Very Irritable* – cannot stand noise. Sneezing – nose stuffed up at night – runs in warm room – must breathe through mouth – *Great Chilliness* not relieved by warmth or bed coverings – lies curled up – so cold dare not move – shivers after drinking – very sensitive to draughts. Later heat with internal chilliness. Sore throat and larynx. Sullen, cross, touchy – even when feverish will not uncover. Hands and face burning – severe headache worse lying on back of head – pain over eyes – cannot stand light – pains in face sinuses affected. Other remedies to consider – Cad-s: Aesc: Caus:

AFTER EFFECTS OF INFLUENZA

Temperature normal in the morning but stays about 99° every evening. Gelsemium 30.

Great debility and chilliness especially if there has been a lot of sweating when ill. China 30.

Depression and nervous debility, sometimes almost suicidal. AUR:30 CAD:30 Scutellaria 30.

General weakness and nerves. Kali-phos:30.

Partially recovers then relapses with hot and cold flushes – sensitive to draughts. Sulphur 12.

Fits of rage, unbearable temper. Influenzium 30.

Vertigo, lassitude, drowsiness. Nat-sal:

After 'flu cough. Coc-c: Kali-s: Pho: Sang:

Loss or partial loss of taste and smell. Mag-m:6. A few doses often sufficient.

General Tonic

Crataegus 1x plus Ferrical (Nelson).

Two tablets Ferrical morning and night and one tablet Crataegus 1x after mid-day meal.

Alfalfa tincture: 10 drops in a tablespoon of water – twice daily.

For those who are prone to cold and influenza every year: Bacillinum Influenzinum 30.

The dose: One tablet every 28 days during the Winter months.

THROAT AND LARYNX

THROAT IN GENERAL
*ACON: Aesc: Ail: AP: Arg-n: Arum-t: BAR-c: *BAR-m: *BELL: Caps: Caus: Gel: *HEP: Jab: KALI-bi: Lac-c: *LACH: LYC: Lys: Merc-c: *MERC-cy: Merc-d: MERC-i-f: MERC-i-r: *MERC: NIT-ac: NUX-v: PHO: PHYT: PULS: RHUS-t: Sul:

ALTERNATING SIDES
ALU: Arn: Coccl: Colo: *LAC-c: Pod: Puls: Sul:

LEFT SIDE
Calc-c: Caus: Diph: Fer: Kali-c: Lac-c: *LACH: Mar: MERC: *MERC-i-r: Naj: Petr: Ph-ac: *RHUS-t: SABAD: SEP: SIL: SUL:

LEFT TO RIGHT
Calc-c: Lac-c: *LACH: *MERC-i-r: RHUS-t: Sabad: Stan:

RIGHT SIDE
AP: BELL: Bry: IGN: Kali-m: *LYC: MERC: Merc-d: MERC-i-f: Phyt: Sang: Stan: Sul: Tarn:

RIGHT GOING TO LEFT
Ap: BELL: Caus: *LYC: *MERC-i-f: Pho: Sang: Sul-ac:

BURNING, SMARTING SCALDED FEELING
Acon: AESC: Ap: *ARS: Ars-io: ARUM-t: Aur: Bar-c: Bell: *CANTH: *CAPS: Carb-ac: *CAUST: *GEL: Hydr: Iris: Kali-bi: Lyc: *MERC-c: Merc-i-f: Merc: MEZ: Nit-ac: *PHOS: *PHYT: SANG: SUL:

COLOUR

BRIGHT RED
*ACON: Ap: *BELL: Fer-p: Caps: Gels: Lyc: Merc: *SUL:

DARK, DUSKY RED
Aesc: AP: *BAPT: *PHYT:

PURPLISH
*AIL: Bapt: Kali-bi: *LACH: Merc: Nux-v: Puls: Phyt:

THICK OR THIN DARK GREY OR BROWNISH BLACK DEPOSIT
*MERC-cy-30: *CALL DOCTOR AT ONCE*

LUMP SENSATION
Hep: IGN: *LACH: Lyc: *NAT-m: Phyt: Puls: Sep:

LUMP SENSATION ON SWALLOWING
BAR-c: Ferr: GELS: GRAPH: LACH: MERC: NAT-m: NUX-v: SEP: Sul:

LUMP SEEMS TO RETURN AGAIN AFTER SWALLOWING
Calc-c: LAC-c: *LACH: RUMX:

SPLINTER OR FISHBONE SENSATION
Arg-n: Hep: Merc-i-f: Nit-ac:

HOT DRINKS RELIEVE
ALUM: *ARS: Calc-fl: CHAM: CHEL: *HEP: *LYC: Nux-v: RHUS-t: Sabad: SPONG: SUL:

HOT DRINKS AGGRAVATE
AP: Calc-c: *LACH: Merc-d: Merc-i-f: Pho: *PHYT:

SWALLOWING SOLIDS RELIEVES
Ign: Lach:

PAIN EXTENDING TO EAR
Arg-n: CHAM: GEL: *HEP: Kali-bi: Kali-m: Lac-c: Lach: *MERC: Merc-d: Nit-ac: Phyt: Sang: Stap:

NECK GLANDS SWOLLEN
*BELL: Hep-s: Kali-bi: *MERC: NUX-v: PHYT: RHUS-t: SUL:

Gargle with freshly squeezed lemon juice at the first indication of a sore throat.
Later PHYT:0 or HYD:0 eight drops to half a glass of water.
For very young children use Rose's Lime Juice neat.

TONSILS IN GENERAL
Bar-c: *BAR-m: *BELL: GUAI: *KALI-m: *LACH: MERC-cy: Merc: *MERC-i-f: *MERC-i-r: *NIT-ac: Phyt: Rhus-t:

CHRONIC ENLARGED TONSILS
*BAR-c: CALC-fl: CALC-p: Lyc: Merc: Merc-i-f: Merc-i-r: Nit-ac: Stap:

CREAMY
Nat-p:

DARK GREY OR BROWNISH BLACK
*MERC-cy: *CALL A DOCTOR AT ONCE*

GREY
*KALI-m: Merc: Merc-i-f: Merc-i-r: Phyt:

GREYISH WITH FIERY RED MARGINS
Ap:

RED – DARK PURPLISH
Aesc: Ail: Bapt: Carb-ac: *LACH: Phyt:

YELLOW LIKE CHAMOIS LEATHER
KALI-bi: Phyt: *RHUS-t:

YELLOW OR WHITE SHINING GLAZED
LAC-c:

TONSILS SUPPURATING
Bell: Hep: Lach: LYC: MERC: *SIL: TARN:

UVULA ENLARGED
*AP: Kali-bi: Merc-c: MERC: Phyt:

UVULA ULCERATED
Kali-bi: Merc-sul-cy:

UVULA WITH YELLOW SPOTS
Nit-ac:

Note KALI-m: has proved very useful in follicular
tonsilitis. The throat looks greyish with white spots
– use the 6x potency every 2 hours.

PAIN LARYNX AND TRACHEA
Acon: *ALL-c: Arg-n: *BELL: Bro: Bry: CAUS:
Dro: DULC: Euphr: Fer-p 2x: GELS: HEP: IOD:
Kali-bi: *LACH: Merc: Mang: Nat-m: NUX-v:
*PHO: PULS: Rhus-t: RUMX: Sele: SPO: Sul:

ROUGH – RAW
Arum: BELL: *CARB-v: Caust: HEP: Keli-io:
MANG: Merc: *NUX-v: *PHO: Puls: *RHUS-t:
RUMX: *SPO: Stan: Sul:

TALKING OR SINGING AGGRAVATES
ACON: Agar: BELL: HEP: *PHO: SPO: Rumx:

TOUCHING AGGRAVATES
ANT-t: Bell: *LACH: *PHO: *SPONG:

WORSE SWALLOWING
BELL: DROS: MERC-c: *SPO: Sul-ac:

PAIN IN TRACHEA
ACON: *BRY: *RUMX: Seneg:

ADENOIDS
AGRAP: CALC-c: *CALC-p: *MERC: *TUB:

CROUP
*ACON: Apis: Brom: *HEP: Kali-bi: Kali-io: Kali-s:
Merc-cy: Pho: *SPO:

Worse Before Midnight
SPO: (sounds like a saw and dry)

Worse Lying and After Midnight
HEP: (Rattling)

Recurrent
CALC-c: *CALC-s: *HEP: PHO:

URINATION

BED WETTING
    *BELL: CALC-c: *CARB-v: *CAUS: Cina:
EQUIS: Ferr: Merc: *PULS: RHUS-t: *SEP: Sil:
*SUL: Tub: etc.

BURNING HOT
    ACO: AP: *ARS: BELL: *BERB: BOR:
*CANTH: Equis: HEP: LYC: *MERC: *MERC-c:
Nat-c: Nit-ac: *NUX-v: SEP: SIL: *SUL: *THU:
etc.

BURNING FROM A CHILL
    ACON:

CHILD CRIES BEFORE URINATING
    ACO: *BOR: *LYC: NUX-v: *SARS:

FREQUENT FROM CATCHING COLD
    DULC: EUP-pur: IP: LYC: Puls:

FREQUENT ONLY IN THE DAYTIME
    Fer: Ham: MAG-m: NAT-m: Psor: *RHUS-t: Staph:

FREQUENT DAY AND NIGHT
    ALY: CALC-c: CANTH: CAUST: COLCH:
*MERC: NAT-m: PLAN: RHUS-t: Sars:

FREQUENT URGING DURING FEVER
    Ant-t: *AP: BELL: PULS:

INEFFECTUAL URGING IN CHILDREN
    *ACON: AP: LYC:

**INEFFECTUAL DESIRE IN NEWLY MARRIED
WOMEN**
    STAPH:

PAINFUL – DIFFICULT IN DROPS
    *CANTH: Cham: EQUIS: *MERC-c: *NUX-v:
Puls: Staph: SUL:

SCANTY
    *AP: *CANTH: Colch: Dig: EQUIS: Graph:
HELL: Op: Rut: Staph:

URGING AFTER COITION
  NAT-p: PH-ac:

DREAMS OF URINATING AND WETS THE BED
  Carb-v: KRE: Lyc: Merc-i-f: SENEG: SEP: Sul:

VOICE

DEEP
  *CARB-v: Colch: *DROS: PHO: POP-c: STAN: SPO: VERB:

FROM COLD DAMP WEATHER
  CARB-v: CAUST: DULC: MANG: RUMX: SIL:

HIGH, PIPING
  ARUM-t: BELL: SPO:

HIGH PITCHED
  (See under "Throat and Larynx".)

HOARSENESS DURING A COLD
  ARS: BRY: *CARB-v: *CAUST: DROS: Fer-p: GEL: KALI-bi: Kalm: MAG-m: *MANG: *MERC: MERC-i-r: NAT-c: Nat-m: NIT-ac: PETR: *PHO: RAN-b: RUMX: SEP: SPIG: *SPONG: TELL:

PAINFUL
  ARG-m: *BELL: BROM: IOD: KALI-bi: *PHO: STAN:

PREVENTING TALKING
  CAUST: MAG-m: *PHO: SPO:

WORSE EVENING
  *CARB-v: *CAUST: GRAPH: KALI-bi: MANG: *PHO: RUMX: SUL:

WORSE MORNING
  ACO: APIS: *CALC-c: *CALC-p: *CAUST: EUPHR: KALI-bi: MANG: NAT-m: NIT-ac: *PHO: SIL: *SUL:

For speakers who have to use their voice a lot 10 drops of Calendula Tincture in half a glass of water makes a soothing gargle. A few doses of Arnica 30 are helpful.

VOMITING

AFTER RICH OR FAT FOOD
  IP: PULS:

AFTER WATER BECOMES WARM IN STOMACH
  *BISM: *PHO: PYRO:

AFTER BEING OVERHEATED
  ANT-c:

CHILD'S VOMIT LIKE CURDS
  AETH: CALC-c:

CHILD VOMITS MILK
  AETH: MAG-c:

DURING INTOXICATION
  NUX-v:

FAINTS AFTER
  ARS: NUX-v:

FROM SMOKING
  IP:

FROM TEETHING
  CALC-c:

IMMEDIATELY AFTER DRINKING A SMALL QUANTITY
  Apoc: *ARS: *BISM: *BRY: *CADM-s: EUP-pf: NUX-v: *PHO: PYRO: Sep: Zn:

ON RAISING THE HEAD
  ARS: *BRY: COLCH: Stram:

RETCHING AFTER VOMITING
  AP: ARS: *COLCH: SEC-c: SEP:

VOMITING BILE WITH A HEADACHE
  BRY: CALC-c: *CHEL: *IP: *IRIS: NAT-s: PULS: *SANG:

VOMITING WITH COLD SWEAT
  ANT-t: *ARS: *CAD-s: CUP-ar: TAB: *VER-a:

VOMITING AND DIARRHOEA
*ANT-t: Ap: ARG-n: *ARS: Bapt: Bor: *CAD-s:
Cam: Cham: Colch: Coloc: Cup: GAMB: IP: IRIS:
Merc: Pho: PODO: Sec-c: Sul: *VER-a:

FORCIBLE
Con: Nux-v: Petr: Sanic: *VER-a:

VOMIT IS WATERY
ARS: *BRY: CAUS: Dros: Tab: *VER-a:

WITH COLIC OR CRAMPS:
CHIN: Coloc: Cup-ar: Iod: NUX-v:

WITH DIZZINESS
See under "Vertigo".

VOMITING DURING PREGNANCY (Morning Sickness)
Anac: Coccl: Ign: *IP: KRE: LOB: Med: Nux-v:
SEP: Sul:

VOMITING WITH PAIN IN ABDOMEN (Slight touch aggravates pain)
Give no medicine or food and call a Doctor immediately.

Should no Doctor be available – give Lachesis 30.

THIRST BEFORE VOMITING
Eup-pr:

THIRST AFTER VOMITING
Sul-ac:

NAUSEA
See under "Sensations".

WOMEN'S MONTHLY PERIOD (Menstruation)

AGGRAVATION BEFORE MENSES
Bov: Bry: CALC-c: Calc-p: Cimic: Coccl: Con: CUP: Hyo: *KALI-c: Kali-m: Kre: Lac-c: *LACH: Lil-t: LYC: Nat-m: Pho: Phyt: *PULS: Sep: Stan: *SUL: VER-a: Vib-o: ZN:

AGGRAVATION BEFORE AND AFTER
BOR: Calc-c: Fer: GRAPH: Kali-m: Kre: LAC-c: *LACH: Lil-t: Mag-c: NAT-m: Pall: Thu:

AGGRAVATION DURING
*AM-c: Arg-n: Bov: Calc-c: Carb-s: Castr: Caus: Cham: Cimic: Coccl: *GRAPH: HYO: Ign: Kali-c: MAG-c: *MAG-m: Nux-m: Nux-v: Pho: Plat: *PULS: Sec-c: STAPH: SUL: ZN:

BEFORE THE PROPER AGE
ANT-c: CALC-c: CALC-p: Carb-v: CAUST: CHAM: Chin: Cocc-c: PHO: PULS: SABI: SIL: Ver-a:

BURNING (Menses)
KRE: SUL:

DAYTIME ONLY (Menses)
CAUST: *PULS:

FAINT (Faints with Menses)
NUX-m: SEP:

FIRST PERIOD DELAYED
Ap: CALC-c: CALC-p: *CAUST: FER: *GRAPH: *KALI-c: MANG: *NAT-m: Polyg: *PULS: *SENEC: SEP: SUL: TUB:

INTERRUPTED, REAPPEARING
AMB: BOV: FER: *KRE: LACH: NUX-v: PHO: *PULS:

IRREGULAR IN TIME AND AMOUNT
Cimic: Coccl: Ign: Iod: Nux-m: SEC-c: Senec: Plat: etc.

MENSES EARLY
Amb: ARS: *BELL: Bor: BOV: BRY: *CALC-c:
CARB-v: Caul: CHAM: COCCL: FER: IP: KALI-c:
MANG: NAT-m: *NUX-v: PHO: *PLAT: RHUS-t:
SABI: etc.

MENSES LATE
*CAUS: *CON: Cup: *DUL: *GRAP: *KALI-c:
LACH: *LYC: *MAG-c: *NAT-m: NUX-m:
*PULS: *SEP: *SIL: *SUL: Vib:

ONLY DURING SLEEP
*BOV: MAG-c:

PAINFUL
*BELL: CALC-c: *CALC-p: *CHAM: *CIMIC:
COCCL: CON: Cup: GRAPH: KALI-c: LACH:
LYC: *MAG-p: Med: NUX-m: PHO: PLAT: PULS:
SEP: SUL: TUB: VER-a: VIB: VER-v: ZN-val:

PALE COLOUR
FER: GRAPH: NAT-m: etc.

SCANTY
*AM-c: *CARB-s: *CON: *CYCL: *DUL:
*GRAPH: Goss: *KALI-c: *LACH: MANG:
MAG-c: NAT-m: *PHO: *PULS: *SUL:

THICK
ARG-n: BELL: CACT: CARB-v: COCCL: FL-ac:
GRAPH: KALI-p: LIL-t: MAG-c: NIT-ac: NUX-m:
PLAT: *PULS: SUL:

THIN
ALUM: BELL: BERB: Bov: DULC: *FER:
*FER-p: GRAPH: LAUR: NAT-m: PHO: *PULS:
SABI: SEC-c: UST:

THIN WITH CLOTS
CHAM: CHIN: FER: SEC-c:

TOO LONG-LASTING
Calc-c: Cup: *FER: Lyc: *NAT-m: *NUX-v: Plat:
Sec-c:

TOO PROFUSE

Ars: Bell: Calc-c: CAUST: CHIN: Croc: Fer: *FER-p: IP: KALI-c: Mel: *NAT-m: Nux-m: NUX-v: PHO: Plat: SABI: Sec-c: Sep: SIL: Stram:

MISCELLANEOUS

ACIDOSIS
Nat-ph:6 is a leading remedy.

ACNE
Calc-p: Kali-brom: Sul-iod:3.

ALVEOLITIS (Dry socket after removal of a tooth)
BOR:6.

ANKLE – sprained
Ruta:6. Arn:12 or Rhus-t:12 may be needed.

ARTERIORSCLEROSIS
Bar-c:30

ATHLETE'S FOOT
Sil:6.

BARBER'S ITCH
Sul-iod:3.

BELLS PALSY (paralysis of side of face)
Caust:12. Expert Homoeopathic advice should be considered.

BONES
To assist bones to knit, Symp:6, three times a day.

BREASTS – Lumps (Mastitis)
Phytolacca 6, three times a day for four weeks, then Conium 6, three times a day for three weeks. Sometimes Pulsatilla if she is that type.

Always under medical supervision.

BRONCHITIS Capillary
One dose of Antimonium tartaricum 10M as soon as possible.

BRUCELLOSIS Recurrent
Hep:30, one a day for twenty days; then Brucella-abortus:30, one a day for three days.

69

BURNS

First treat for shock with Arnica 200, then soak a pad of gauze with Urtica urens tincture, 20 drops to a cupful of water, cover with a pad of cotton wool and bandage.

Keep the gauze moist with the solution but do not remove gauze.

Give internally Urtica urens 30, repeat when pain returns.

For Second Degree Burns as above, only use Hypericum tincture externally and give Causticum 6 internally 2 hourly.

When healing is well advanced use Calendula ointment.

CANCER (Pains from)

Epithelioma, of face, nose or lip
Hydrastis 6, one tablet three times a day.

Rectal
Alum: Ruta 6, Hydrastis 6: Nit-ac: Sep:
Mammae
Con:6, Hydrastis:6, Carb-an:6, Sang:6
Antrum
Aur: Symp:6
Bone
Aur-iod: Phos: Symp:6
Stomach
Ars:6, Bism:3, Cad-s:6, Condur: Hydr:6, Kreos: Pho: Plat-mur:
Tongue
Radium-brom:30
Cervix
Carb-an: Hydr: Iod: Kreos: Thuja: Lapis-albus 30.

The following have been found to relieve the general pains.

Apis: Ars: Cad-s: Euphorb: Hydr: (all in 6 potency).

These are only a few of possible remedies that might be required. Symptoms and conditions of aggravation or amelioration should be studied in the Repertory. According to Continental sources, a dose of Cadmium-sulph:30 every 12 or 20 days has a remarkable effect on the general health of a sufferer from cancer.

CARBUNCLE
Anthracinum 30 every 4 hours.
Tarentula Cub. 12 every 4 hours.

CHICHEN-POX
Rhus-tox:
The main remedy.

Ant-tart:
Tardy eruption or blueish rash or if associated with bronchitis.

Merc-sol:
If vesicles suppurate.

CHILBLAINS
The hands and feet should always be protected from the cold, also the ears in severe weather.

Externally paint Tamus tincture on affected parts.

Most painful from cold
Agar:6

Worse when near a fire or heated
Pul:6

For those with damp cold feet
Calc-c:6

Warm patients liable to skin complaints
Sul:6

If splits or chaps occur
Petr:6

Should suppuration take place
Hep-s:30

CHOLERA

Camphor 30
>Patient very cold but won't be covered.

Cuprum-met:30
>Severe cramps, wishes to be covered.

Veratrum-alb:30
>Cold sweats with violent vomiting and diarrhoea. The forehead is particularly wet.

CHOLERA MORBUS
ANT-t: (nausea but relief after vomiting).

COLIC
Dios 3: better by stretching and moving. Colo 6: better by bending, worse motion.

CONSTIPATION

Chronic
>BRY:6, Collin:3 (with bleeding piles), Grap: *NUX:30, Op:30, Plb: *SUL: Ver-a:3.

Lack of:– roughage in the diet, daily exercise and attending to nature's call at once, and the use of aluminium kettles and pans are often the main causes.

Stools difficult though soft
>*ALUM:12, Chin: HEP: Ign: *NUX-m:6, Plat: Psor: Pul: SEP: Sil: Staph:

Urging Abortive
>Anac: Lyc: Nat-m: *NUX-v:30, Pul: Sep: Sil: Sul:12.

Absence of Urging
>Alum: *BRY: Graph: Hyd:1x, *OP:30.

The Constitutional Remedy, i.e. the remedy that covers the whole person, will usually cure constipation as well as any other complaints.

Small quantities of bran added to a breakfast cereal is helpful, plus black treacle.

The use of wholewheat bread is, however, preferable.

CORNS
Ant-c:6

COUGHS
Dry
Aco: Bell: Bry: Nux-v: Pho: Rumx:

Loose
Calc-c: Kali-bi: Kali-c: Puls: Sep:

Worse cold drinks
Calc-c: Hep: Sil: Sul: Ver-a:

Better cold drinks
*CAUS: Coc-c: Cup: Tab:

CRAMP
Nux-v: Cupr: Led: Cupr-a:

CROUP
Aconite
From exposure to cold wind, develops croup the same evening in the first sleep.

Spongia
From exposure to cold winds a day or so before.

Both develop croup usually before midnight.

If Aconite only partially controls, Spongia follows beyond midnight.

Dry cough, sawing respiration, no rattling.

Hepar-sulph:
If croup returns next morning or evening – or with rattling. The child is chilly.

Calcarea-sulph:
The child is too hot and kicks off the blankets.

73

DIPTHERIA
(Should be treated only by an experienced Homoeopathic doctor.)
Merc-cy:30.

Post-diptheric paralysis
Gels:

DIVERTICULITIS
*NUX-v:30, Aloes:3, Ver-a:3.

A difficult condition: these remedies may be tried. Diet is very important.

Too much roughage may cause irritation and pain once the condition is confirmed.

DYSLEXIA
Try Lyc:6 three times a day for three weeks.

ELBOW – Tennis or blow on
Ruta:6.

EYES
Lids Twitching
Agar:6

Glandular Cysts
Thuja:30

Squint
Gels:6 three times a day for two weeks.

Blepharitis
Eyelids sticking together in the morning – Jacaranda.

Detachment of Retina
Naphthalinum

These conditions should be treated by an experienced Homoeopathic physician.

FEET ODOUR
Bar-c: GRAPH: *KALI-c: Nit-ac: Puls: SIL: *SEP: Thuja:

FELON OR WHITLOW
Hep:30

"FROZEN" SHOULDER
Aco 12: Caus 6: Lachn 6:

FUNGUS – around the nails
Keep the fingers dry and apply Gentian Violet.

GALLSTONE COLIC
Often relieved by BELL: or Bry: Coloc: Dio: Leptandra, as indicated.

Other possibles – Chin: Berb: Chel:

If septic symptoms arise, give one dose of Sepia M.

GLANDULAR FEVER (Mononucleosis)
Ailanthus-glan:6 three times a day for 10 days. I have never known this to fail.

Cytomegalovinus
Similar to Glandular Fever though less severe.

Like German Measles virus, it is capable of infecting the foetus.

Ailanthus-glan:6 as above.

Recurring Glandular Fever
Tuberculinum-bovum (high potency).

I usually give one 30, then seven days later one 200 and seven days after that one M. A possible alternative is Bar-c:30.

GLAUCOMA
Pho:

GONORRHOEA
Main Remedies
Arg-n: Acon: *CANN-sat: (Copaiv-sep: in females), Canth: Gels: Naphthalin: Merc-c: Merc-v: Nat-s: Pul: Tussilago: Petros: Sul: *THUJA:

Acute Inflammatory Stage
*ACON: Arg-n: *CANN-sat: Canth: Caps: *GELS: Petros.

Symptoms should decide the choice.

HAIR
Ringworm – Dulc:6.

HEART
Worse after sleep – cough – anxiety – difficult respiration – cannot lie with head low – SPONGIA.

General Heart Tonic
Crat-oxy: tincture. 5 drops in tablespoon of water 3 times a day after food. Slow acting.

HERPES LABIALIS
(Pearl-like blisters on lips and round the mouth.)

Rhus-t: Nat-m:

HICCOUGHS
Niccolum: Nux-v:

HOME-SICKNESS
Caps:30

HYPERTENSION (High Blood Pressure)
Should be treated by an experienced Homoeopathic doctor.

Patient's constitutional remedy or Eel Serum 6 one tablet daily for a week has been found effective, or Lycopus 3 one dose daily until improvement.

IMPETIGO
Ant-c:12

Impetigo Contagiosa
Arum-tr:200 daily for three days.

INFLUENZA
Main remedies are Baptisia, Bryonia, Causticum, Eupatorium-per: Gelsemium, Rhus-tox: (Refer to Part 2).

JOINTS (Fluid in after injuries)
  Ruta 30 three times a day.

KIDNEY STONE (also Nephritis)
  Give Polygonum-sagittatum Mother Tincture two drops in water night and morning – reduce with progress.

  Berberis 10M repeated will often cause a small stone to pass.

  Should be under the care of a Homoeopathic doctor.

LEG ULCERS IN THE AGED
  Externally
    Calendula ointment once a day.

  Internally
    If from a fall Arnica 200, twice a day for two days.

    With varicose veins – Hamamelis 6, twice a day.

    With great pain – Fluoric acid 30, three times a day.

    As much rest as possible, with feet up.

    Hydrastis 3 sometimes helpful. Also Ars: Kali-bi: Sil:

LIVER AND RIGHT HYPOCHONDRIUM
  Aco: Alo: Ars: Aur: Bell: Berb: *BRY: Calc-c: *CHEL: Chin: Chio: Dio: Hyds: Iris: Kali-c: Lach: *LYC: Mag-m: *MERC-s: Nat-s: *NUX-v: Pho: Pod: Sep:

LOCOMOTOR ATAXIA
  Alum: Kali-p:

LUMBAGO
  Aco: Rhus-t: (Calc-fl: if Rhus-t: fails), Ant-t: with retching.

  NUX-v: has to sit up to turn in bed.

MALARIA RECURRENT
*NAT-m: Ars: Eup-pf: Ip:

MEASLES suspected, *Aconite*.

PULS:
Dry mounth but seldom thirst

Gelsemium
If indicated.

Sul:
Rash slow to come out – purplish appearance.

Measles Cough
Scilla 12.

Euphrasia
Streaming burning tears.

Ferr-ph:
With unduly high temperature.

GERMAN MEASLES
Puls:

MENIERES DISEASE
Nat-sal:6, China: Chin-s:

(Coming on during sleep or after sleep – Lach:6).

MENINGITIS CEREBRAL
(Must be under medical care).

Acute Stage
Aco: or Bell: (if from a blow Arn:)

After effusion
Bry: (with shrill cries in sleep Apis:3).

Later in patients subject to eruptions, Sul:

Tubercular
One dose Bacilinum 30.

After the fever has subsided Zinc-met:6 may be required.

MISCARRIAGE
Give a few drops of Viburnum-op:12. This often stops the haemorrhage and causes expulsion of secundine.

MORNING SICKNESS of Pregnancy
Ipec: Nux-v: Sep:

MUMPS
Jaborandi
is the main remedy.

Puls:
If girl's breasts swell or boy's testicles swell.

Carbo-veg:
Will bring the trouble back to its original place.

NEVER WELL SINCE

Chicken Pox:	Vaicella 30.
Diphtheria:	Diphtherium 30.
German Measles:	Rubella 30.
Influenza:	Influenzinum 30.
Measles:	Morbillinum 30.
Mumps:	Parotidunum 30.
Scarlet Fever:	Scarletinum 30.
Smallpox:	Variolinum 30.
Typhoid:	Typhoidinum 30.
Whooping Cough:	Pertussin 30.

Give three doses in one day at intervals of eight hours. There may be some reaction a few days later but on no account repeat.

PARALYSIS OF SINGLE PARTS
*CAUS: Gels: Nux-v:

PHLEBITIS
Viper: Ham: Pul: (after childbirth).

Externally
Ham: Tincture.

PILES

*AESC:(often with backache). *ALO:(loose stool), Calc-fl:30, CARB-v:(windy), Caus: *COLLIN (bleeding only on pressure), Graph: HAM:(bleeding), Hypr: Kali-c: Lach: Lyc: Merc-i-r: *MUR-ac: *NIT-ac: *NUX-v: Paeon: Pho: Pul: Sep: *SUL:

A little bran helps.

Postpartum Haemorrhoids – Kali-c:

Externally – Hypercal Ointment.

PROSTRATE

Thuja: Puls: Kali-iod:

(Sensation as if sitting on a ball – Canabis-ind: Chimaphila-umb:)

Difficult passing urine *SABAL-ser: Solidago-vig:

In old man, chronic enlargement – Arg-mur: Arg-nit: *FER-pic: Euphr:6x,

PURPURA HAEMORRAGIA

CROT-h:(blood almost black and stringy). LACH:(blood dark – worse after sleep). PHOS:(blood bright red, restless).

SCARLET FEVER

Bell:

SCLEROSIS MULTIPLE

At first sign: Kali-p:

Possibles: Aur: Aur-mur: Arg-n: Pho: Plumb: Zinc-ph:

SHINGLES (Herpes Zoster)

Rhus-tox:
Great itching and tingling of the skin.

Ranum-bulb:
Vesicles in clusters filled with thin acrid fluid.

Mezereum:
If caught early.

80

SLEEPWALING
   Sil:

SMALLPOX

Antimonium-tart:
   Before or at the beginning of eruptive stage, also
   when eruption fails.

Variolinum 30
   Great thirst – sometimes diarrhoea – limbs numb –
   violent headaches and pains.

Must be under medical care.

Hydrastis
   Is the main remedy where lips, mouth, throat,
   bright red, dry and burning.

   After suffering with ulceration – Cham:

Malignant Scarlet Fever
   Ailanthus:(Rash blueish).

   Face swollen – pustules dark, faintness, great
   prostration, worse at night.

Malandrium 30
   Said to be a preventative.

Thuja
   Follows Antimony-tart: well.

SCIATICA
   Almost any remedy may be necessary. The following
   are a few possibles:
   Bry:(worse movement), Bufo: Gnaphalium 6(with
   numbness), Iris: Kali-i-iod:3(has to walk about at
   night), Mag-ph:30(better heat), Nux-v: Lyc: Rhus-t:12
   (better after moving a little), Telurium: Colocynthis:12
   (extends from hip down the back of the thigh to
   behind the knee), Phytolacca:6(pains run down the
   outer side of the thigh), Kali-bic:(better leg flexed).
   Dios:3(right side better if kept still).

SINUSES

See under **Nose** in Part 2.

STINGS

Insects Ledum 12 if severe every few minutes.

Wasp and Bee Apis 30, also every few minutes if severe. Otherwise every half hour for a few doses.

If the part is cold or numb then Ledum is indicated.

STIFF NECK

Aco:12, Caus:6, Lachn:6.

TEETH

Hypr:30 before extraction. Arn:30 after.

Dentures hurt gums – Arn:

TEETHING

If baby is very cross CHAM:30 – crush two tablets between two spoons and dissolve in three tablespoons of cold water – give a teaspoonful every ten minutes.

If there is no sign of rage, just sobbing, give Puls:6 in the same way.

TOOTHACHE

Gumboil

Hep-s:6. When discharging Sil:6.

In a decayed tooth

Merc-s:6.

In an open cavity

Insert cottonwool soaked in Plantago Tincture.

Worse from cold drinks and food

Calc-c:6, Merc:6, Nux-v:12.

Worse from warmth in general

Cham: Merc-s: Puls:

Worse from cold and heat

Calc-ph: Lach: *PLANTAGO 3.

The Plantago can be given every fifteen minutes for a few doses.

WAKEFUL CHILDREN

Sleep during day and play and dance at midnight in their cot.

Cypripedum 6.

WHOOPING COUGH

Carb-veg:
When suspected.

Drosera 30
Just one dose, is the main remedy or Dros:6 after each vomit or paroxym.

Cough returns with every cold with offensive expectoration. Sanguinaria 6.

Coccus-cacti 3 sometimes required. Also Spong:

WRIST SPRAINED

Ruta:6.

REFERENCE TABLES

ANTAGONISTIC REMEDIES

ALL-CEP: – Aloe: Scilla:

ACETIC ACID: – Bov: Caus: Nux-v: Ran-b: Sars:

AMMONIUM-CARB: – Lach:

APIS: – Rhus-t:

BAPTISIA: – Influenzinum.

BELLADONNA: – Dulc:

BENZOIC ACID: – Copaiv:

CALC-C: – Nit-ac: Bar-c: Sul:
Do not follow after Kali-bi: and Nit-ac:

CAMPHOR: – Kali-n:

CANTHARIS: – Cof:

CARBO-VEG: – Kreasot:

CAUSTICUM: – Acetic-ac: Cof: Colo: Kali-n: Nux-v: Pho:

CHAMOMILLA: – Zinc:

CHINA: – Dig: Selen:

COCCULUS: – Cof:

COFFEA: – Canth: Caus: Coccul: Ign:

COLOCYNTH: – Caus:

DIGITALIS: – Strop: Chin:

DULCAMARA: – Bell: Lach: Acet-ac:

IGNATIA: – Calc-c:

KALI-BI: – Calc-c:

KALI-NIT: – Cam: Caus: Ran-b:

LACHESIS: – Am-c: Dul: Nit-ac: Sep:

LYCOPODIUM: – Nux-m:
    (Sul: follows after but not before).

MERCURY: – Phyt: Lach: Sil:
    (Lach: after Calc-c:)

NITRIC ACID: – Lach: Nat-m:

NUX-MOSCHATA: – Lyc: Nux-v: Pul: Rhus-t: Sil:
Squilla:

NUX-V: – Acetic-ac: Caus: Ign: Nux-m: Zin:

PHOSPHORUS: – Caus:

RANUNCULUS-BULB: – Acetic-ac: Kali-n: Staph: Sul:

RHUS-TOX: Apis:

SARSAPARILLA: – Acetic-ac:

SELENIUM: – Chin:

SEPIA: – Lach: Bry:

SILICA: – Merc: Nux-m:

STAPHYSAGRIA: – Ran-b:

SULPHUR: – Nux-m: Ran-b:

ZINCUM: – Cham: Nux-v:

Fuller details of remedies that follow well and antidotes
can be found in Dr J. H. Clarke's "Clinical Repertory".

PAINS IN GENERAL
Refer to various organs like chest, throat, liver, head, etc.

CRAMPING PAINS
  Cuprum, Cuprum-ars: Colocynth, Magnesium-phos:

BURNING PAINS
  Arsenic: Canthar: Capsic: Phos: Sul-ac:

WITH COLDNESS (sensation)
  Calc-c: Ars: Cistus: Helod:

WITH COLDNESS (objective)
  Camph: Secale: Verat-alb: Heloderma.

FULLNESS (sensation)
  Aescul-hip: China: Lyc:

EMPTINESS (sensation)
  Coccul: Phos: Sepia:

BEARING DOWN
  Bell: Lil-tig: Sep: etc.,

WANDERING OR ERRATIC
  Kali-bi: Kali-s: Pul: Lac-c: Mang-ac: Plat:

BRUISED SORENESS
  Arn: Bapt: Eupat-perf: Pyrogen: Ruta: Bellis:

CONSTRICTION
  Cact-gr: Colocy: Anacard:

PROSTRATION OR WEARINESS
  Gel: Pic-ac: Phos-ac: Stan:

NUMBNESS
  Acon: Cham: Plat: Rhus-t:

ERRATIC PAINS
  Lac-c: Pul: Tub-bov:

SENSITIVENESS TO PAIN
  Aco: Cham: Cof:

SENSITIVE TO TOUCH
  Chin: Hep: Lach:

BONE PAINS
  Aur: Asaf: Eup-per: Merc: Mez:

STICKING OR STITCHING PAINS
    Bry: Kali-c: Squilla:

PULSATING OR THROBBING
    Bell: Glon: Melilotus: Nat-m:

HAEMORRHAGES (passive)
    Ham: Secale: Crot-h: Elaps:

HAEMORRHAGES (active)
    Fer-ph: Ipec: Phos:

EMACIATION
    Iod: Nat-m: Lyc: Sarsa:

LEUCOPHLEGMASIA
    Calc-c: Graph: Capsicum

CONSTITUTIONS (Psoric)
    Sul: Psor: etc.,

CONSTITUTIONS (Sycotic)
    Thuj: Nit-ac: Medorrhinum:

CONSTITUTIONS (Syphilitic)
    Kali-iod: Merc: Syphilinum: Mez:

BLUE SWELLINGS
    Lach: Pul: Tarant-cub:

TEARING PAINS AND RAWNESS
    Caust:

HAEMORRHAGES

All symptoms must be taken into consideration.

Ipecacuanha
    Bright red, profuse with heavy breathing and nausea.

Aconitum
    Active, bright with great fear or anxiety.

Arnica
    From injuries – bodily fatigue or physical exertion.

Belladonna
    Blood hot – throbbing carotids, congestion to head.

Carbo-Veg.
    Almost entire collapse – face pale – wants to be fanned.

Hamamelis
    Very dark and clotted – veins enlarged and sore to touch – bruised feeling.

China
    Great loss of blood, ringing in the ears, faintness.

Crocus
    Blood clots in long dark strings.

Ferrum
    Partly fluid – partly solid – very red face or red and pale alternately.

Hyoscyamus
    Delirium and jerking and twitching of muscles.

Lachesis
    Blood decomposed – sediment like charred straws.

Crotalus   *Elaps*   *Sul-ac*
    Black fluid blood – the first and last from all outlets.

Nitric-ac.
    Active haemorrhages of bright blood.

Phosphorus
    Profuse and persistent even from small wounds or tumours.

Platinum
    Partly fluid and partly hard black clots.

Pulsatilla
    Intermittent haemorrhages.

Secale
    Passive flow in feeble cachectic women.

Sulphur
    In psoric constitutions and if other remedies fail.

Viper 200
    Bleeding from nose with vertigo.

RHEUMATISM
Rheumatism would require a book to itself, so here are just a few tips.

WORSE WARMTH
    Bry: Led: Phos: Phyt: Puls: Thuja:

BETTER COOL
Led: Puls:

BETTER WARMTH
Ars: Caust: Colch: Coloc: Lyc: Merc: Nux-v: Rhus-t: Sul:

WORSE COLD WET
Arn: Colch: Dulc: Rhus-t: Verat:

WORSE COLD DRY
Acon: Bry: Caust: Hep-s: Nux-v:

BETTER WET OR WORSE DRY
Asar: Bry: *CAUST: Hep-s: Kali-c: Nux-v: Sep: Spong:

BETTER WARM WET
Caust: Hep-s: Nux-v:

WORSE MOTION
*BRY: Fer-p: Lac-can: Led: Salicyl-ac: Sticta: CHEL:

BETTER MOTION
Cham: Dulc: Rhod: *RHUS-t: *PULS:

WORSE WET
Puls: Verat: (Compare "Cold Wet").

SHIFTS RAPIDLY
Kalm: Lac-can: *PULS: Kali-bic:

NUMBNESS WITH PAIN
Acon: Cham: Puls:

WORSE JAR
Arn: *BELL: *BRY: Hep-s: Led: Nux-v: Rhus-t:

WORSE TOUCH
Arn: *BELL: Bry: Cham: *COLCH: Hep-s: Led: Med: Nux-v: Puls: Rhod: Rhus-t:

UNAFFECTED BY CHANGE OF WEATHER EXCLUDES
Dulc: Nux-m: Phos: Ran-b: Rhod: Rhus-t: Sil: Tub-bov:

NOT AFFECTED BY DAMPNESS EXCLUDES
Calc-c: Merc: Nux-v: Ruta:

The Constitutional Remedy should not be overlooked.

A FEW "DONT'S"

ACONITE
Never give in blood poisoning such as scarlet fever or typhoid conditions where there is stupor and purplish skin.

AILANTHUS-GLAN:
Discontinue in scarletina when eruption begins to fade.

ANACARDIUM-ORIENTAL
Don't repeat too often.

ANTIMONY-TART:
Discontinue if eruption like smallpox is produced.

ARNICA
Is contra-indicated where there is an excessive coagulability of the blood.

BELLADONNA
Is not indicated in continuous fevers such as typhoid – it will do harm.

CALCAREA-CARB:
Not to be repeated in persons of very advanced age.

CAUSTICUM
Can produce warts as well as cure them. (Should not be taken over a long period).

KALI-CARB:
Start low.

KALI-SALTS
Do not use in high fevers.

LACHESIS
To be used with care in very high potency.

LYCOPODIUM
Avoid the 200 potency.

NAT-MUR:
Give Nux-v: if headache is produced.

PHOS:
Very dangerous high in advanced T.B. (can start haemorrhage).

SILICA
Use with caution in lung T.B. – not high.

SULPHUR
Give in high potency at long intervals.

THUJA
Should not be repeated often. One dose of 200 best.

VERATRUM-VIRIDE
Don't use in weak hearts or in pneumonia.

ABBREVIATIONS

THE 25 REMEDIES MARKED WITH TWO ASTERISKS
ARE A SUGGESTED LIST FOR THE BEGINNER.

THOSE WITH ONE ASTERISK ARE ALSO VERY
USEFUL.

THE REMAINDER COVER A LARGE FIELD AND
CAN BE ACQUIRED WHEN NECESSARY.

These abbreviations are as used by Dr C. M. Boger.

Abro:	Abrotanum.
**Aco:	Aconitum napellus.
*Aesc:	Aesculus hippocastranum.
Aeth-c:	Aethusa cynapium.
*Agar:	Agaricus muscarius.
Agn-c:	Agnus castus.
Ail:	Ailanthus.
All-c:	Allium cepa.
Alo:	Aloe.
*Alum:	Alumina.
Amb:	Ambra.
Amm-c:	Ammonium carbonicum.
Anac:	Anacardium orientale.
Anthrac:	Anthracinum.
*Ant-c:	Antimonium crudum.
**Ant-t:	Antimonium tartaricum.
**Api:	Apis mellifica.
Aral-r:	Aralia racemose.
Arg-m:	Argentum metallicum.
*Arg-n:	Argentum nitricum.
**Arn:	Arnica montana.
**Ars:	Arsenicum album.
Arum-t:	Arum triphyllum.
Aur:	Aurum metallicum.
Bacil:	Bacillinum.
**Bap:	Baptisia.
*Bar-c:	Baryta carbonica.
Bar-m:	Baryta muruatica.
**Bell:	Belladonna.
*Bellis:	Bellis perennis.

Benz-ac:	Benzoicum acidum.
*Berb:	Berberis vulgaris.
*Bism:	Bismuthum.
Bor:	Borax.
Bov:	Bovista.
Brom:	Bromium.
**Bry:	Bryonia alba.
Cact:	Cactus grandiflora.
Cad:	Cadmium metallicum.
Cad-s:	Cadmium sulphuratum.
Calad:	Caladium.
*Calc-c:	Calcarea carbonica.
*Calc-fl:	Calcarea fluorata.
Calc-i:	Calcarea iodata.
*Calc-p:	Calcarea phosphorica.
Calc-s:	Calcarea sulphurica.
Calend:	Calendula.
†Camp:	Camphor tincture.
Cann-s:	Cannabis sativa.
**Canth:	Cantharis.
Caps:	Capsicum.
Carb-a:	Carbo animalis.
**Carb-v:	Carbo vegetablis.
Card-m:	Carduus marianus.
Caul:	Caulophyllum.
*Caus:	Causticum.
**Cham:	Chamomilla.
*Chel:	Chelidonium.
*Chin:	Cinchona officinalis.
Chin-s:	Chininum sulphuricum.
*Cimic:	Cimicifuga racemosa.
Cina:	Cina.
Cistus:	Cistus canadensis.
Clem:	Clematis erecta.
*Coccl:	Cocculus indicus.
Coc-c:	Coccus cacti.
*Coff:	Coffea cruda.
Colch:	Colchicum.
Collin:	Collinsonia.
**Colo:	Colocynthis.
Con:	Conium.
Crat-oxy:	Crataegus oxyacantha.
Croc:	Crocus sativus.
Crotal-h:	Crotalus horridus.

Cupr:	Cuprum metallicum.
Cupr-a:	Cuprum aresenicosum.
Cyl:	Cyclamen.
Dig:	Digatalis.
Dios:	Dioscorea villosa.
*Dros:	Drosera rotundifolia.
*Dulc:	Solanum dulcamera.
Ecchin:	Ecchinacea angustfolia.
Elap:	Elaps corallinus.
Equis:	Equisetum.
Eucal:	Eucalyptus globulus.
*Eup-pf:	Eupatorium perfoliatum.
Eup-pur:	Eupatorium purpureum.
Eupho:	Euphobium officunarum.
Euphr:	Euphrasia.
Ferr:	Ferrum.
**Ferr-p:	Ferrum phosphoricum.
Ferr-pic:	Ferrum picricum.
Fluor-ac:	Fluoricum acidum.
**Gels:	Gelsenium.
Gent-l:	Gentiana Lutea.
*Glon:	Glononium.
Gnaph:	Gnaphalium.
*Graph:	Graphites.
Grat:	Gratiola.
Guaiac:	Guaicum.
Gunp:	Gunpowder.
*Ham:	Hamamelis.
Hell:	Helleborus niger.
**Hep:	Hepar sulphuris.
*Hyd:	Hydrastic cenadensis.
Hyo:	Hyoscyamus niger.
**Hypr:	Hypericum perfoliatum.
**Ign:	Ignatia.
Indm:	Indium.
Infl:	Influenzinum.
Iod:	Iodum.
**Ip:	Ipecacuanha.
Iris:	Iris verisocolor.
Jac:	Jacaranda.
Just:	Justica adhatoda basaka.
**Kali-bi:	Kali bichromicum.
Kali-c:	Kali carbonicum.
*Kali-i:	Kali iodatum.

Kali-m:	Kali muriaticum.
*Kali-p:	Kali phosphoricum.
Kali-s:	Kali sulphuricum.
Kalm:	Kalmia latifolia.
Kre:	Kreosotum.
Lac-c:	Lac canimum.
*Lach:	Lachesis.
Lachn:	Lachnanthes tinctoria.
Lath-s:	Lathyrus savitus.
Laur:	Laurocerasus.
**Led:	Ledum palustre.
Lil-t:	Lilium tigrinum.
Lob:	Lobelia inflata.
*Lyc:	Lycopodium clavatum.
Lyss:	Lyssin.
*Mag-c:	Magnesia carbonica.
Mag-m:	Magnesia muriatica.
Mag-p:	Magnesia phosphorica.
Mang:	Manganum.
Med:	Medorrhinum.
Meli:	Melilotus alba.
*Merc-c:	Mercurius corrosivus.
*Merc-cy:	Mercurius cyanatus.
Merc-d:	Mercurius dulcis.
*Merc-i-fl:	Mercurius iodatus flavus.
*Merc-i-r:	Mercurius iodatus ruber.
**Merc:	Mercurius solubilis.
Merc-v:	Mercurius vivus.
Mez:	Daphne mezereum.
Mill:	Millefolium.
Mur-ac:	Muriatucum acidum.
Murx:	Murex purpurea.
Naph:	Naphthalinum.
Nat-c:	Natrum carbonicum.
*Nat-m:	Natrum muriaticum.
*Nat-p:	Natrum phosphoricum.
*Nat-s:	Natrum sulphuricum.
Nat-sal:	Natrum salicylicum.
*Nit-ac:	Nitricum acidum.
Nux-m:	Nux moschata.
**Nux-v:	Nux vomica.
Op:	Opium.
Orig:	Origanum.
Osm:	Osmium.

Paeon:	Paeonia.
Pall:	Palladium.
Pareir-b:	Pareira brava.
Parf:	Paraffine.
Paris:	Paris quadrifolia.
Pass-i:	Passiflora incarnata.
*Petr:	Petroleum.
Petros:	Petroselinum.
Phel:	Pellandrium aquaticum.
**Pho:	Phosphorus.
Ph-ac:	Phosphoricum acidum.
*Phyt:	Phytolacca.
Pic-ac:	Picricum acidum.
*Plant:	Plantago major.
Plat:	Platina.
Plumb:	Plumbum metallicum.
*Pod:	Podophyllum peltatum.
Poly:	Polygonum sagittatum.
Pop-c:	Populus candicam.
Pru-s:	Prunus spinosa.
Pso:	Psorinum.
**Puls:	Pulsatilla nigricans.
*Pyro:	Pyrogenium.
*Quilla:	Quillaya saponaria.
*Ran-b:	Ranunculus bulbosus.
Raph:	Raphanus sativus.
Rat:	Ratanhia.
Rham:	Raminus californica.
Rho:	Rhododendron.
**Rhus-t:	Rhus toxicodendron.
Rob:	Robina.
*Rumx:	Rumex crispus.
*Rut:	Ruta.
*Sabad:	Sabadilla.
Sabal:	Sabal serrulata.
Sabi:	Sabina.
Samb:	Sanbucus nigra.
Sang:	Sanguinaria canadensis.
Sanic:	Sanicula aqua.
Sar:	Sarasapilla.
Scil:	Scilla maratina.
Sec-c:	Secale cornutum.
Sele:	Selenium.
Seneg:	Senega.

*Sep:	Sepia.
*Sil:	Silica.
Solid:	Solidago viragoaurea.
Spig:	Spigelia.
**Spong:	Spongia.
Squ:	Squilla maritima.
Stan:	Stannum.
*Staph:	Staphysagria.
Stram:	Stramonium.
Stroph:	Strophantus hispidus.
Sul-ac:	Sulphurosum acidum.
*Sul:	Sulphur.
Symp:	Symphytum.
Tab:	Tabacum.
*Tarn:	Tarentula cubensis.
Tarx:	Taraxacum.
Tell:	Tellurium.
Tereb:	Terabinthina.
Ther:	Theridian curassavicum.
*Thuja:	Thuja occidentalis.
Tub-bov:	Tuberculinum bovum.
*Urt-u:	Urtica urens.
Val:	Valeriana.
*Ver-a:	Verat album.
Ver-v:	Verat viride.
Verb:	Verbascum thapsus.
Vib-op:	Viburnam opulus.
Vin-m:	Vinca minor.
Vio-o:	Viola odorata.
Vio-t:	Viola tricolor.
Vip:	Vipera communis.
Zn:	Zincum.
Zn-v:	Zincum valerianicum.

†*Note* Camphor tincture pills should be kept in a separate drawer from other remedies as they are apt to make them ineffective.